A Strategic Guide to Continuing Professional Development for Health and Care Professionals:
The TRAMm Model

Full the full range of M&K Publishing books please visit our website:
www.mkupdate.co.uk

A Strategic Guide to Continuing Professional Development for Health and Care Professionals: **The TRAMm Model** (2nd Edition)

Deb Hearle and
Sarah Lawson

A Strategic Guide to Continuing Professional Development for Health and Care Professionals:
THE TRAMm Model

Deb Hearle & Sarah Lawson

ISBN: 9781910451243

First published 2016, 2nd edition published 2020

All rights reserved. No part of this publication may be reproduced, stored in a retrieval system, or transmitted in any form or by any means, electronic, mechanical, photocopying, recording or otherwise, without either the prior permission of the publishers or a licence permitting restricted copying in the United Kingdom issued by the Copyright Licensing Agency, 90 Tottenham Court Road, London, W1T 4LP. Permissions may be sought directly from M&K Publishing, phone: 01768 773030, fax: 01768 781099 or email: publishing@mkupdate.co.uk

Any person who does any unauthorised act in relation to this publication may be liable to criminal prosecution and civil claims for damages.

British Library Cataloguing in Publication Data
A catalogue record for this book is available from the British Library

Notice

Clinical practice and medical knowledge constantly evolve. Standard safety precautions must be followed, but, as knowledge is broadened by research, changes in practice, treatment and drug therapy may become necessary or appropriate. Readers must check the most current product information provided by the manufacturer of each drug to be administered and verify the dosages and correct administration, as well as contraindications. It is the responsibility of the practitioner, utilising the experience and knowledge of the patient, to determine dosages and the best treatment for each individual patient. Any brands mentioned in this book are as examples only and are not endorsed by the publisher. Neither the publisher nor the authors assume any liability for any injury and/or damage to persons or property arising from this publication.

Disclaimer

M&K Publishing cannot accept responsibility for the contents of any linked website or online resource. The existence of a link does not imply any endorsement or recommendation of the organisation or the information or views which may be expressed in any linked website or online resource. We cannot guarantee that these links will operate consistently and we have no control over the availability of linked pages.

To contact M&K Publishing write to:
M&K Update Ltd · The Old Bakery · St. John's Street
Keswick · Cumbria CA12 5AS
Tel: 01768 773030 · Fax: 01768 781099
publishing@mkupdate.co.uk
www.mkupdate.co.uk

Designed and typeset by Mary Blood
Printed in England by McKanes Printers, Keswick

Contents

List of tables	vi
List of figures	vii
About the authors	viii
Acknowledgements	viii
Preface	ix
1 What is continuing professional development (CPD) and why do we do it?	1
2 What counts as CPD activity?	11
3 Taking responsibility for CPD: Changing mindsets	31
4 Recognising your strengths and developing your preferred learning style	51
5 Introduction to the **TRAMm model**	59
6 How do you plan and disseminate your CPD? **TRAMm Station T: TELL**	71
7 How do you record your CPD plans and activities? **TRAMm Station R: RECORD**	93
8 How can you apply your CPD? **TRAMm Station A: APPLY**	119
9 How do you keep track of your CPD? **TRAMm Station M: MONITOR**	129
10 How do you measure your CPD? **TRAMm Station m: mEASURE**	145
11 Conclusion	165
References	171
Index	177

List of tables

Table 1.1	HCPC registered professional bodies and website addresses	4
Table 1.2	International CPD requirements	7
Table 3.1	Examples of learning and development frameworks	38
Table 3.2	Business case for CPD activity	47
Table 5.1	Suggestions for entries included in the stations of the TRAMm Model stations	65
Table 7.1	Example of a learning contract template	97
Table 7.2	The TRAMm Tracker: a brief overview	104
Table 7.3	The TRAMm Trail: A brief overview of the stations and suggested content	106
Table 8.1	Sample intervention evidence chart	124
Table 9.1	SWOT analysis: Sally and her profile for promotion	141
Table 10.1	Definition of service user versus context	147
Table 10.2:	Useful HCPC information	149
Table 10.3	Types of evidence	150
Table 10.4:	Referencing anecdotal evidence	159

List of figures

Figure 3.1 Stages of successful professional development	35
Figure 5.1 The TRAMm Model stations	64
Figure 5.2 Sally's first attempt at completing a TRAMm Tracker	70
Figure 6.1: Sally's amended TRAMm Tracker	91
Figure 7.1 Example of a mind map	96
Figure 7.2 Blank TRAMm Tracker page 1 Overview of the HCPC standards and TRAMm stations	110
Figure 7.3 Blank TRAMm Tracker page 2	111
Figure 7.4 Blank TRAMm Trail	112
Figure 7.5 Strategic TRAMm Trail	113
Figure 7.6 Sally's updated TRAMm Tracker	115
Figure 7.7 Sally's TRAMm Trail Planning for rotation into neurorehabilitation	116
Figure 7.8 Sally's TRAMm Trail: TRAMmCPD	117
Figure 8.1 Sally's updated TRAMm Tracker	127
Figure 8.2 Sally's updated TRAMm Trail rotation into neurorehabilitation	128
Figure 9.1 Sally's updated TRAMm Tracker	143
Figure 9.2 Sally's TRAMm Trail: Career Development Planning	144
Figure 10.1 Sally's updated TRAMm Tracker	163
Figure 10.2 Sally's TRAMm Trail: Service development	164

About the authors

Deb Hearle
Senior Lecturer and Head of Health Professions Cardiff University; MSc Interprofessional Studies (Health), Dip COT, PGCE (HE), FHEA, Dip ISM

Deb is an occupational therapist and an experienced educator and manager. She has been teaching healthcare students (including aspects of professional development) at both undergraduate and postgraduate level for 30 years. She runs study days and postgraduate courses which contribute to CPD. She also accredits professional courses (alongside the Health and Care Professions Council) where CPD is a requirement. Deb is a member of the TRAMmCPD development team and explored CPD engagement as part of her doctoral studies.

Sarah Lawson
Occupational Therapist, PhD Candidate, BSc (Hons) Occupational Therapy; BSc (Hons) Health and Social Welfare

After spending eight years working as a community occupational therapist in social care, Sarah began her PhD building underpinning evidence for the TRAMm Model. She is researching engagement in, and application of CPD and how this relates to TRAMmCPD. Sarah is a member of the TRAMmCPD development team and leads on website development as well as managing TRAMmCPD's social media presence.

Acknowledgements
Our thanks to Roe Morris who was part of the original TRAMmCPD development team and contributed to the first edition of this book.

Preface

Welcome to this new, updated edition of your strategic guide to continuing professional development (CPD). This second edition includes new chapters, wider professional policy guidance updates and results from our ongoing research exploring professional development within health and social care. New information has been included to reflect changes to the TRAMm Model – most significantly, the change to TRAMm Station A (from Activity to Apply) to reflect the importance of using and applying new learning in practice to benefit yourself, the people who access your service and others.

The original chapter about the types of CPD activities you choose to engage in has been retained but moved outside the TRAMm Model (Chapter 2). New material includes an additional chapter on changing mindsets about CPD and how to create opportunities for learning and development, despite limited resources in the current economic climate (Chapter 3). There is also an expanded chapter about CPD engagement and what it means to be actively involved in your own learning and development (Chapter 2), with updated evidence on exploring your preferred styles of learning (Chapter 4).

CPD is an essential component of today's working practice for all professionals involved in health and social care. It is a core aspect of clinical governance and is closely linked with quality monitoring and improvement. Professional bodies have produced guidelines to support and direct the professional development of nurses and allied health professionals (AHPP 2003, Broughton & Harris 2019). When there is significant investment in CPD (whether individually or via organisational policy), the individual feels valued and happy in their work and their quality of practice is shown to improve (Van den Broeck, Vansteenkiste et al. 2008, Schaufeli & Bakker 2004). In contrast, when CPD is given limited attention, this has been shown to correlate with work-related stress and burnout, resulting in increased staff sickness, absence and subsequent decreased productivity (Van den Broeck, Vansteenkiste et al. 2008, Schaufeli & Bakker 2004). This has been recognised in the NHS Long Term Plan (2019) which includes increased investment planned for improving development opportunities for staff.

Although all health and social care staff are familiar with the term 'CPD' and are aware of its requirements, there are many different ideas about what constitutes CPD and the ways in which health professionals are expected to demonstrate their personal and professional development.

Since the introduction of the Health and Care Professions Council (formerly the Health Professions Council) in 2002, the profile of CPD for health and care professionals has risen significantly. There are now many workplace processes and procedures that are not only designed to monitor and measure performance but also to identify training needs. Such processes include preceptorship, supervision, appraisal/professional development review and clinical audit. Health and care professionals are commonly expected to complete professional development portfolios and there is guidance available on how to record your progress. However, there is little explanation of the reasons for undertaking CPD or advice on how professionals can fully embrace it as an integral part of their practice, rather than as something that has to be done solely to meet professional and organisational requirements.

What is the purpose of this book?

There is a growing demand for knowledge and specialisation, which requires health and care students and professionals to adopt varied and innovative approaches to learning. This, together with the drive to embrace and integrate new technologies, helps to facilitate the active engagement rather than passive participation (Hearle & Lawson 2019) of students and professionals in CPD. TRAMmCPD is a package that brings all these aspects of learning together. It provides a toolkit to encourage a more strategic approach to your personal and professional development. It consists of a model illustrating the requirements for evidencing your engagement in CPD, with a set of tools to help you:

- Plan and record your activities
- Apply and disseminate your CPD
- Monitor and measure your progress.

After an introduction to CPD, an exploration of the types of activities you might engage in, how to think differently about CPD and a section helping you to identify your strengths and preferred learning styles, the book follows the stages (depicted as stations) of the TRAMm Model, namely: Tell (T), Record (R), Apply (A), Monitor (M) and measure (m). It discusses their integration, illustrating the core principles by means of a concurrent case study. Your own learning needs will provide the main focus, enabling you to develop a full profile that will meet the requirements of CPD as the chapters progress. At the end of each chapter, there are opportunities to reflect on your learning and apply theory to practice through questions and tasks.

Who is this book for?

As will become evident, this book is primarily (but not exclusively) aimed at those professionals registered with the Health and Care Professions Council (HCPC) who, as part of their biennial re-registration process, must undertake and evidence CPD. The HCPC do not 'approve' particular CPD activities or CPD schemes but encourage registrants to use whatever they find helpful and relevant to their development.

There are currently 15 professional groups registered with the HCPC: arts therapists, biomedical scientists, chiropodists/podiatrists, clinical scientists, dieticians, hearing aid dispensers, occupational therapists, operating department practitioners, orthoptists, paramedics, physiotherapists, practitioner psychologists, prosthetists/orthotists, radiographers, and speech and language therapists (HCPC 2019a).

This book is designed to be accessible for all levels, from health and care students to experienced practitioners. In addition, the text may be useful for associated support workers and other healthcare professional groups who are also required to undertake CPD, such as doctors, pharmacists, optometrists, social workers, nurses and midwives. Some aspects of the book will also be useful for professionals outside the health and care professions, who are required to undertake and evidence CPD. The primary focus of this book is health and social care professionals in the United Kingdom (UK). However, some key issues presented will be relevant to other professionals and/or to practitioners overseas. Although this handbook is designed to build knowledge and skills by logical progression through all the chapters in sequence, you can also access individual chapters or sections as required.

Authors' note

In December 2019 a new regulatory body, Social Work England (SWE), was established for social workers in England.

We are making final editorial changes to this book in April 2020, when the world is under global restrictions due to Coronavirus (COVID-19). The Health and Care Professions Council (HCPC) have suspended the Continuing Professional Development (CPD) audits for Physiotherapists, Art Therapists and Dietitians that were due to take place in 2020. The HCPC have also set up a temporary register for final-year students who have completed all clinical learning outcomes so that they can enter the health and social care workforce in order to meet the unprecedented demands being placed on health and social care services.

Within practice and education, health and care professionals are being expected to upskill in new areas and at a speed never before experienced, as we progress towards a new state of 'normal'. There is currently little evidence related to COVID-19 on which to base our practice, and health and care professionals are continuing to adapt to new information as it becomes available. CPD therefore continues, and has in fact never been more important, as people are expected to learn and develop in new ways.

This book refers to a variety of face-to-face CPD activities which have now either been postponed or moved online using virtual technologies. However, regardless of the medium in which CPD activities are carried out, the principles of the TRAMm Model remain the same: to be most effective we need to Tell others; Record and Apply what we have learnt; Monitor our progress; and measure the impact.

1

What is continuing professional development (CPD) and why do we do it?

This chapter defines CPD and explains why it is important. It introduces the key professional requirements – particularly those of the Health and Care Professions Council (HCPC), which are discussed in depth. A brief overview of professional contacts in the UK is also presented, as well as some useful international links for anyone considering coming to the UK or working outside the UK.

The chapter concludes by examining the potential impact of CPD on a person's personal and professional development and their practice. This will be illustrated with a case study, which will continue through all the chapters (to illustrate the use of the TRAMm Model). There are tasks at the end of the chapter, to encourage you to consider what you already know about CPD and the implications of the HCPC standards and professional guidelines. You will also be asked to reflect upon the impact your CPD has on your practice.

What is CPD?

The Allied Health Professions Project (AHPP) (2003, p. 9) defines CPD as

> a range of learning activities through which health professionals maintain and develop throughout their career to ensure that they retain their capacity to practise safely, effectively and legally within their evolving scope of practice.

This definition has been adopted by the HCPC (2017a) for the purpose of regulation.

CPD is an ongoing process that usually begins as soon as an individual completes their qualification for their chosen career. In the field of health and social care, it applies to practitioners, educators, managers and researchers. In forward-thinking organisations, it can also be applied to any member of staff, including support, administrative, domestic and technical staff. In most health and social care professions, students are also encouraged to commence their CPD when they begin their course of study, by using and developing a professional portfolio (see Chapter 7). This helps them develop ways of planning and structuring CPD records for their future careers and lifelong learning. CPD and lifelong learning are interlinked as fundamental aspects of improving the knowledge and skills needed to work effectively and contribute to a sense of personal fulfilment (Broughton & Harris 2019). Lifelong learning continues across the whole lifespan and is considered to underpin CPD.

The principles of CPD also apply to many professions outside health and social care, including teaching, surveying, engineering and the law. Each profession has its own CPD requirements, ranging from a mandatory course or minimum required CPD hours and/or CPD points to an outcome-based approach where the emphasis is on impact.

Many practitioners do not have a strategic personal development plan and the process and practice of CPD is often misunderstood. Some may attend workshops, courses or professional conferences (whether or not the learning fits their career and learning objectives), in the belief that they are thereby meeting their CPD obligations. For most professions, CPD can cover many types of learning – both formal and informal – and increasingly involve the use of social media and virtual technologies. However, it should always be undertaken in a considered way in order to be meaningful and meet its aims.

Why undertake CPD?
CPD: A mandatory responsibility

The term 'Continuing Professional Development' has been used for many years. However, until the introduction of clinical governance in the UK in 1998, it was not given much importance. Clinical governance was instigated in the National Health Service (NHS) in order to guide the improvement of practice (DH 1998). Scally and Donaldson (1998, p. 61) described it as

> a system through which NHS organisations are accountable for continuously improving the quality of their services and safeguarding high standards of care by creating an environment in which excellence in clinical care will flourish.

Between 1990 and 1995, at the Bristol Royal Infirmary, 35 babies died unnecessarily and dozens were left brain-damaged (DH 2002). The associated scandal provided the impetus for the introduction of clinical governance and the subsequent focus on CPD. In social care, cases such as those of Victoria Climbié in 2000 and Baby P in 2007 stimulated this discussion and led to the instigation of further quality assurance mechanisms. Before 1998, CPD was mostly undertaken by those who were motivated to develop themselves both personally and professionally. Those with lower aspirations could therefore hold back progress in service delivery. However, following the introduction of clinical governance, it was no longer acceptable for health and care professionals to refrain from further development after they had qualified. The need to continuously update knowledge and skills was elevated in status from desirable to expected (Scally & Donaldson 1998).

Scally and Donaldson (1998) highlighted the importance of organisations valuing employees and their professional development, as these employees would be the future leaders of change. They considered that if people in the organisation felt valued, they would strive to make the organisation successful by delivering a high-quality service that ultimately benefited those in their care. This was based on evidence from those deemed to be successful organisations and has been supported by Strong (2009).

Despite changes in government and the NHS, the concept of clinical governance has remained constant. For this reason, there has been growing acknowledgement of the value of CPD and it is now considered to be an important factor in quality improvement, staff retention and a core responsibility of the health and social care professional. Today, all qualified health and social care staff are required to undertake CPD and, in many instances, it is a prerequisite for professional registration.

In the UK, health and social care mandatory requirements and standards are set by regulatory bodies appointed by the Government, such as the HCPC, the Nursing and Midwifery Council (NMC), the General Medical Council (GMC), or country-specific Social Care Councils. Specific requirements depend upon the particular professional group and in some cases (such as social care) these also differ across England, Northern Ireland, Scotland and Wales. For example, in Wales social care staff (apart from occupational therapists) register with Social Care Wales (SCW), previously Care Council for Wales (CCW), and also need to provide evidence of CPD every three years. In Scotland the regulatory body is the Scottish Social Services Council (SSSC), and in Northern Ireland it is the Social Care Council (NISCC).

CPD: A personal and professional responsibility

Although the mandatory requirements described above are of central importance, they are not the only reasons for undertaking CPD. Evidence also shows that we should all see CPD as an essential part of our working lives – for both personal and professional reasons.

Professional education programmes and codes of conduct emphasise our professional responsibility to provide the highest quality of care to service users, even in the absence of mandatory requirements. In order to do this, we must continually develop our skills, based on evidence regarding which interventions work well and which do not, or require special considerations for maximum impact. The NHS Staff Council (2009) found that staff who felt valued (through the provision of professional development opportunities) were likely to demonstrate increased levels of satisfaction and motivation and were therefore more likely to continue working for an organisation. This suggests that, when any CPD is undertaken, staff integrate their learning and skill acquisition into the organisation and help to develop high-quality care together. Another indirect, positive consequence of this is safer and more effective patient care (RCN 2007).

There are also health benefits from undertaking CPD. Strong et *al.* (2003) found that supervision, one method of facilitating CPD, can help to increase job satisfaction, effectiveness and clinical reasoning, while at the same time preventing stress and burnout (see Chapter 7). In organisations such as the NHS, there is a high prevalence of staff absence due to work-related stress

(HSE 2019). This suggests that individual and organisational investment in CPD can also help to reduce these potential health consequences of stress.

This book is written for all HCPC-registered professionals. The principles may apply to anyone who is interested in formalising their professional development, particularly those from healthcare backgrounds. The next section of this chapter will outline specific documented expectations for those registered by the HCPC.

How do you demonstrate CPD?

For health and social care professionals, regulation is undertaken by the HCPC, who stipulate that all registered professionals must demonstrate CPD. At present, 15 professions are regulated by the HCPC (HCPC 2019a). Each one has its own professional body, which provides further support for CPD and has its own HCPC 'Standards of Proficiency'. These standards include some generic elements, which apply to all registrants, as well as some profession-specific elements. The *Standards of Conduct, Performance and Ethics* (HCPC 2016) and the five Standards for CPD in *Continuing Professional Development and Your Registration* (HCPC 2017a) apply to all HCPC regulated professions (HCPC 2019a). The 15 professional groups and their websites are listed in Table 1.1.

Table 1.1 HCPC registered professional bodies and website addresses

Profession	Professional body and website (all accessed 19 February 2020)
Art therapists	British Association of Art Therapists https://www.baat.org/
Biomedical scientists	Association of Biomedical Healthcare Scientists https://www.ibms.org/home/
Chiropodists/Podiatrists	College of Podiatry https://cop.org.uk/
Clinical scientists	Association of Clinical Scientists http://www.assclinsci.org/acsApplicants/acsBodies.aspx
Dietitians	The Association of UK Dietitians https://www.bda.uk.com/
Hearing aid dispensers	British Society of Hearing Aid Audiologists http://www.bshaa.com/
Occupational therapists NB: In 2017 the College of Occupational Therapists was awarded Royal status and became the Royal College of Occupational Therapists	Royal College of Occupational Therapists https://www.rcot.co.uk/

Operating department practitioners	College of Operating Department Practitioners *https://www.unison.org.uk/at-work/health-care/representing-you/unison-partnerships/codp/*
Orthoptists	British and Irish Orthoptic Society *http://www.orthoptics.org.uk/*
Paramedics	College of Paramedics *https://www.collegeofparamedics.co.uk/*
Physiotherapists	Chartered Society of Physiotherapists *http://www.csp.org.uk/*
Practitioner psychologists	British Psychological Society *http://www.bps.org.uk/*
Prosthetists/Orthotists	British Association of Prosthetists and Orthotists *http://www.bapo.com/*
Radiographers (Diagnostic/Therapeutic)	Society of Radiographers *http://www.sor.org/*
Speech and language therapists	Royal College of Speech and Language Therapists *http://www.rcslt.org/*

The HCPC has developed generic CPD standards which require registrants to record their current and relevant activities and ensure learning is transferred into practice to benefit the service user (HCPC 2017a). Every time you renew your registration, you need to confirm that you continue to meet the following standards (HCPC 2017a, p. 5):

1. Maintain a continuous, up-to-date and accurate record of your CPD activities

2. Demonstrate that your CPD activities are a mixture of learning activities relevant to current or future practice

3. Seek to ensure that your CPD has contributed to the quality of your practice and service delivery

4. Seek to ensure that your CPD benefits the service user

5. Upon request, present a written profile (which must be your own work and supported by evidence) explaining how you have met the standards for CPD.

According to the HCPC (2017a, p. 7), this means the following:

1. You must keep a chronological record of your CPD, in whatever format is most convenient for you (e.g. TRAMm Tracker and Trail).

2. You must make sure your CPD is a mixture of different kinds of activities – not just one kind of learning – and that it is relevant to your work. It could be relevant to your current role or to a planned future role or to the future direction of the organisation in which you work.

3. You should aim for your CPD to improve the quality of your work. This may not always be achieved (due to factors beyond your control) but you should always intend your CPD activities to influence and have a positive impact on your practice.

4. You should aim for your CPD to benefit service users; you may not be able to ensure that this happens every time, but you should try to develop practice that clearly benefits the people with whom you work. Depending on where and how you work, this might include your service users, your team or your students (see Table 10.1).

5. If selected for audit, you will need to send a CPD profile (which must be your own work and supported by evidence) to show how you have met the standards (see Chapter 10). Should this profile be incomplete, it may be returned to you for further work. If you do not comply with this request, you will usually be removed from the register – unless your non-compliance is due to 'unavoidable circumstances', in which case you may be allowed to defer (HCPC 2017a, p. 14).

However, it is important to note that these are current HCPC requirements. These could change in the future and it is therefore advisable to refer to the HCPC website (https://www.hcpc-uk.org/) for the most up-to-date information.

For other health and care professionals in the UK, regulatory bodies such as the Nursing and Midwifery Council (NMC) and the General Medical Council (GMC) set out their own standards for CPD. To further emphasise the importance of CPD for the health and care professions, a joint document outlining five guiding principles for CPD and lifelong learning has been developed by a range of health and care stakeholders (Broughton & Harris 2019). This document outlines the responsibilities for you, your employer and wider systems in relation to CPD, which it suggests is everybody's responsibility.

Regulation has been helpful in increasing the significance of CPD for both staff and organisations, encouraging staff to undertake and record CPD with reference to its impact on service users (HCPC 2017a). However, although the HCPC audit highlights measurement against standards of CPD, it may not clearly demonstrate impact on practice. The biennial review also means that people may be 'strategic' about their practice and recording of CPD, rather than making it an integral part of their work.

TRAMmCPD (Hearle, Lawson & Morris 2016) has been developed as a framework with a set of tools to encourage a more thoughtfully strategic and integrated approach to CPD.

International requirements for CPD

Requirements differ from country to country, regarding visas, registration, qualifications to work, language proficiency and CPD. Table 1.2 provides some useful links if you are considering working inside (or outside) the UK as part of your professional development. It may also be useful to contact your own professional body, or that of the country you are planning to work in, for advice.

Table 1.2 International CPD requirements

Country	Useful weblinks (all accessed 19 February 2020)
Australia/Canada/Europe/United States/New Zealand/UK	Visa information is available at: https://www.emigrate2.co.uk/
Australia	Australian Health Practitioner Regulation Agency (Ahpra) governs the operations of the national boards, each board has its own standards and provides guidance. Information available at: https://www.ahpra.gov.au/Education/Continuing-Professional-Development.aspx
Canada	Health Canada provides information and guidance: https://www.canada.ca/en/health-canada/services/health-care-system/health-human-resources/strategy/internationally-educated-health-care-professionals.html Check with your professional body for CPD or Continuing Professional Education guidance (CPE)
Ireland	Information available at: http://www.citizensinformation.ie/en/moving_country/moving_to_ireland/working_in_ireland/ CORU is the multi-professional regulator that provides CPD guidelines: http://www.coru.ie/
South Africa	The Health Professions Council of South Africa is the regulatory body for 12 professional boards. Information is available at: http://www.hpcsa.co.za/ Their professional CPD guidance is available at: https://www.hpcsa.co.za/?contentId=0&menuSubId=18&actionName=Core%20Operations
The United Kingdom (UK)	Passport and living abroad information: https://www.gov.uk/browse/abroad Visa and immigration information: https://www.gov.uk/browse/visas-immigration The HCPC, the regulatory body for health and care professionals in the UK offers information and guidance and sets the Standards for CPD (HCPC 2017a): https://www.hcpc-uk.org/registration/getting-on-the-register/international-applications/

cont.

United States of America (USA)	States across America have different mandatory requirements which range from no requirements to a set number of hours, units (or a mixture of the two) over a period of time.
	USA government information about visas and work is available at:
	https://www.usa.gov/
	The Department of Homeland Security has information about obtaining permanent resident status available at: https://www.uscis.gov/greencard
	Check your professional body for more guidance and information regarding CPD requirements in individual US states.

How do you undertake and demonstrate CPD?

In the past, CPD relied on the individual collecting a series of certificates or points to show that a course had been attended and a specified amount of CPD undertaken. Although there are many free courses available which can be a valuable way of helping you to develop personally and professionally, such courses are not the only means of undertaking CPD, and Chapter 2 explores some options in more detail.

It should also be remembered that simply attending a course or workshop does not in itself constitute CPD. The CPD is how you use and apply what you have learnt, and how you evidence this learning. In the next section we introduce you to our case study practitioner, Sally. We will revisit Sally in future chapters to illustrate how TRAMmCPD might help you engage in CPD. Although Sally is an occupational therapist, her learning experience applies equally to any of the HCPC registered professions.

Case study: Introducing Sally

Sally is an occupational therapist registered with the HCPC. She has been working for seven months, after qualifying a year ago. She is currently in a Band Five post in community mental health, following six months in orthopaedics. She will move into her third rotation on the neurological rehabilitation ward in five months' time.

Sally has just completed her first review as part of her preceptorship programme and knows she must undertake some CPD in the coming year. She is aware that there is a conference coming up in two months' time so, having gained permission from her manager, she registers to attend. Attendance is free but her manager has allowed her to take the time off work and has agreed to give her funding of up to £200 for travel and accommodation.

Sally arrives at the conference and glances at the programme, which looks complicated. She decides to tag along with her friend who is attending a seminar that will last for the first morning. It is in the same building and is next to the coffee room where she is currently, so this seems to be the most sensible option. At lunch she meets a group of friends with whom she went to university and soon realises that she has missed the start of the next set of presentations. She decides to have a wander around the poster display and then go to the exhibition, where she collects information and freebies from the exhibitors' stands. At the next coffee break she hears that there is a session on social media that she is interested in, so she goes to that.

At the end of the social media session, Sally thinks she has done everything she was supposed to do and therefore ticks off CPD on her appraisal objectives. She has attended a conference, gone to some sessions, seen posters and collected loads of free information. She is not too keen on doing the same tomorrow but she needs to stay in order to get her certificate of attendance. She then heads back to the hotel.

In the hotel Sally unpacks her conference bag. Amongst the free pens and leaflets, she finds the conference programme. She looks at the timetable for the following day and notices a seminar on stroke rehabilitation during the morning, which she thinks would be worth attending. Nothing interests her in the afternoon sessions so she decides to wait and see which sessions her friends are going to. The following day Sally attends the stroke seminar as planned and finds it useful. She realises how much more she is enjoying the second day of the conference and wishes she had been more organised the previous day. At lunch, her friends are discussing their afternoon sessions and Sally decides to tag along with them.

Is Sally engaging in CPD? According to the HCPC, Sally has attended several learning activities, which may have helped her learn some new things, but:

- How could she prepare differently, to make the most of future CPD opportunities?
- How could her manager have encouraged her to prepare more effectively?
- How is Sally going to demonstrate that she has a continuous and up-to-date record of her CPD activities? (See Chapter 7, HCPC Standard 1.)
- How will Sally demonstrate that she has undertaken a mixture of learning activities? (See Chapters 2, 5 and 10, HCPC Standard 2.)
- In a year's time, how will Sally remember what she did and what she learnt? (See Chapters 7 and 10, HCPC Standards 1 and 2.)
- How will Sally show that this activity has contributed to the quality of her practice and service delivery? (See Chapters 7, 8 and 10, HCPC Standards 3 and 4.)
- How will her manager know what she has learnt from attending? (See Chapters 6–10, HCPC Standard 3.)
- How will Sally's colleagues benefit from covering for her while she is away? (See Chapter 6 and 8, HCPC Standards 3 and 4.)
- How will the organisation Sally works for benefit from her CPD? (See Chapters 6 and 10, HCPC Standards 3 and 4.)

This book will explore ways in which TRAMmCPD can help you address these aspects and meet the HCPC standards for CPD, whatever your profession, working situation and experience.

Tasks

The following tasks ask you to consider what you already know about CPD and encourage you to find out more about the requirements and support available to you:

1. Read the Principles of Continuing Professional Development and Lifelong Learning in Health and Social Care (Broughton & Harris 2019) and consider how they relate to you and your practice.
2. If you are a HCPC registered health and care professional, read the HCPC CPD and your registration (HCPC 2017a) to familiarise yourself with what is expected of you.
3. If you are not a HCPC registered professional, you can still use TRAMmCPD but ensure that you are aware of the requirements of your own regulatory body.
4. Explore your own professional body website and see what resources they offer to guide and support CPD.
5. Reflect on the ways in which your CPD is currently contributing to your practice.
6. Read Chapter 2 to discover more about the types of activities which may count towards your CPD.

2

What counts as CPD activity?

This chapter discusses the types of activities that can be considered as **CPD and how to maximise their impact. Individuals often engage in activities that contribute towards their professional development without realising they are undertaking CPD – for instance, learning from the advice of colleagues, being on a committee, undertaking long-arm supervision, researching current projects, reading a journal, external examining and attending conferences. This chapter gives guidance on how to choose the most appropriate type of CPD activity for your needs. It is not intended to be a full 'how to guide'. Rather, it will help you consider and select the most appropriate forms of activity and investigate their use and potential as part of your self-directed learning.**

Tasks at the end of the chapter will encourage you to consider which of the activities you have already undertaken have had the most impact on your CPD and reflect on why this has been the case.

What do we mean by CPD activity?

In this context, 'activity' refers to something undertaken in order to learn. CPD often begins with an activity, although this is not always best practice, as explained in Chapter 6, where we have illustrated the importance of beginning by thoughtfully planning your own professional development needs.

For the HCPC (2017a), any activity that enables you to learn and develop can potentially be considered to contribute to your CPD. Numerous types of activities can be included as part of professional development, such as:

- Liaising with other professionals/agencies
- Training activities beyond mandatory and specialist training
- Learning from colleagues
- Undertaking your own informal research
- Reading journals or joining journal clubs
- Shadowing/secondments/rotation

- External examining
- Gaining accreditation, approval or revalidation
- Undertaking reflection
- Pursuing further education
- Doing project work
- Getting involved with your professional body
- Being an active member of a specialist section or interest group
- Undertaking preceptorship (or its equivalent)
- Attending conferences or courses
- Engaging in workshops
- Listening to podcasts.

The HCPC (2017a) provides a list of ideas for possible CPD activities under the following headings: Work-Based Learning, Professional Activity, Formal/Educational, Self-Directed Learning and Other. They expect registrants to make professional judgements about the appropriateness, context and frequency of activities in order to meet the minimum CPD standards. For the purpose of this chapter, these headings have been considered and reflected in sub-groups as follows: Formal activities, Informal activities, Professional/External activities, Professional support, Training, Informal support, Social media, Self-directed learning and Reflection. Remember that all activities can be useful CPD but you need to consider the context in which you are going to apply them, as the learning outcomes will vary according to the context and the individual.

The decision as to where your activities fit within the stations of the TRAMm Model is entirely your own and may depend on the context in which they are undertaken and your own preferences. These lists are not exhaustive, and you may undertake many other activities that you decide to use as evidence for your CPD.

Why do we need to undertake learning activities and how do we choose what to do?

Although the main reason for CPD highlighted by HCPC (2017a) is to protect the public by ensuring that registrants are fit for practice and meet minimum standards, it is important for professionals to think *beyond* minimum standards. For practice to develop, practitioners must consider which activities will help them to develop higher-quality practice and the additional skills they may need to influence quality provision (such as higher-level communication skills, entrepreneurial and management skills, research skills and the ability to teach others). As a professional, you should not only be undertaking the activities required to do your current job, but also those that will enable you to do it to the best of your ability or make it possible for you or others to undertake additional tasks in the future.

Researchers have found evidence of the benefits of undertaking CPD, despite the challenges of attributing improved performance outcomes to a particular event or activity. For example, in a study of physiotherapists' perceptions of the outcomes of CPD (Gunn & Goding 2009) participants acknowledged that there had been significant positive effects from CPD undertaken. Positive outcomes (such as development in professional competence, management of patients and those with complex problems, an increased ability to build productive therapist–patient relationships through improved communication skills and increased levels of understanding) led to them feeling valued.

This links with Dall'Alba's theory of 'embodiment' (Dall'Alba & Barnacle 2005) where a greater understanding of practice is thought to result in enhanced professional ability and a more holistic approach. Although these were reported outcomes of CPD, Dall'Alba and Barnacle (2005) acknowledged that it was often difficult to attribute these factors directly to CPD and our challenge as health and care professionals is how we demonstrate this link clearly. For those who really engage in CPD, there may be many individual benefits (see Chapter 3).

There are many different types of activities that can enable you to develop, both professionally and personally, and provide evidence of your learning. Chapter 4 explores ways to identify your strengths and preferred learning styles, with some reasons why this may be important when considering your choice of CPD activity. The following section gives some examples of the wide variety of activities you could undertake, together with suggestions for measuring their success and how they may contribute to your CPD.

Formal activities

Formal activities, such as education, research and project work, are important and valuable. They not only help to further your own professional development and lead to possible promotion, but they can also contribute to the advancement of the profession and the growth of evidence-informed practice in service delivery.

Research

Research skills, like any other aspect of practice, cover a very wide spectrum. At one end of the scale, there are undergraduate projects or small-scale service evaluations; at the other end, there are sophisticated systematic reviews and large-scale, funded, randomised, controlled trials. Whatever form it takes, research is everybody's business, from professionals using supporting evidence within their everyday practice, to those undertaking large-scale research studies and everyone in between. Its importance is reflected in current pre-registration education of health and care professionals which requires all students and trainees to understand the importance of using and undertaking research in practice.

Health and care professionals from all backgrounds must utilise research but not all are required to be researchers themselves. However, we all have a responsibility to ensure that practice and overall service delivery are evaluated so that we learn from best practice and strive to develop areas that need further improvement (see also 'project work' below).

In order to participate in research, you do not need to secure the funding or be the principal investigator ('project lead'). In fact, for early-stage researchers, this is often not possible, particularly for larger projects. Instead, you may form part of the overall team contributing to one small part of the project, such as data collection. You can also attend formal training to develop your own skill in this area.

If you are a more advanced researcher, you may already know how to put a bid together. If not, seek help from your local research and development board, professional body, university or local library service or from university colleagues. A good site to explore is the Health Research Authority (HRA), at www.hra.nhs.uk (last accessed 21.2.2020).

Project work

Although project management has been mentioned in research above, it covers many different aspects, including small-scale service development projects, introducing new policies and undertaking specific quality improvement projects. Projects are being initiated all the time, particularly in the health and care environments, but it can be difficult to get involved in leading or being part of the project team unless you actively seek such opportunities.

Small-scale project management is a great way to develop your overall management skills, and if your project is successful it can provide evidence to use for your CV and for applications for promotion. If you are new to project management, there are also short courses that may help you to develop these skills. These courses may be provided on an in-service basis or externally (for instance, by your organisation or your local university). If you have managed small projects before but wish to take on something a little more complex, formal training could include courses such as PRINCE 2 methodology.

Formal educational study

There are a great many formal educational opportunities such as higher education degrees, Open University courses, distance learning modules and skills-based courses. For further information, investigate opportunities available at local universities or further education colleges, or search online for distance learning courses.

How can you measure the success of your formal learning opportunities?

For most formal learning opportunities, providing some sort of evidence or measurement for what you have done is an easy process, as there is usually a clear outcome such as a certificate, project report or qualification. This is one reason why these types of opportunities are a popular form of CPD.

Research provides CPD by:
- Expanding your knowledge and skills in relation to the research process
- Encouraging you to read/critique articles and other literature on current practice, then develop conclusions to be disseminated and integrated into practice
- Developing data collection and analysis skills, which may be transferred into practice (e.g. narrative analysis or interviewing and service evaluation or improvement projects)
- Developing project management skills
- Helping to increase your understanding of the roles of other professionals (especially if working on a collaborative project) and thus providing opportunities for greater networking and more effective team working in practice
- Enabling you to ensure that your interventions are utilising the most up-to-date, relevant research to benefit the people who access your service.

Project work provides CPD by:
- Developing your skills and understanding of change management
- Giving you experience of team working
- Helping you learn about financial management
- Possibly helping you to understand the roles of other professionals (if the project work is interdisciplinary)
- Giving you experience of managing a team, including leadership, delegation and negotiation
- Familiarising you with project planning and developing objectives
- Improving your advanced report writing skills
- Enabling you to develop applications for funding.

Formal educational study provides CPD by:
- Offering you many benefits, which very much depend on the type of learning undertaken and may include any of the above suggestions.

Mapping formal opportunities to the TRAMm Model stations can be easy if the activity is fairly short and simple. For a long course or project, you may decide to split the activity into sub-sections because you learn something different at each stage. (For instance, in a degree course you may undertake a management module that teaches you one set of skills, and then undertake a research module that provides you with others.) Formal educational study can be easily measured in terms of outcome. However, additional aspects (such as reflection or evaluation of how effectively your learning has been applied in practice) may need further explanation. An example of this could be a research project that has demonstrated the effectiveness of a new intervention. Research is often undertaken in controlled circumstances so your additional measurement may evaluate how this has been implemented in normal day-to-day practice.

Informal activities

Less formal activities include worked-based learning and journal clubs.

Work-based learning

Work-based or workplace learning 'refers to CPD that is stimulated by and occurs through participation in workplace activities' (Lloyd, Pfeiffer et al. 2014, p. 1). Put simply, working and learning occur simultaneously, and work-based learning is considered essential for high-quality care, especially when there is limited funding for formal training. This is becoming an increasingly popular approach to CPD, as reflected by the development of apprenticeships across health and social care.

Work-based learning does not usually require any formal application process, and it can provide very clearly focused development of knowledge and/or skills specifically related to your workplace. These can include activities such as shadowing (learning alongside an expert colleague), secondments (periods of time spent working within another role, department or organisation while maintaining your main post), rotations, in-service training (training provided by or within the organisation) and mentoring/teaching colleagues. Work-based learning may also include e-learning activities (such as e-modules) or it can be linked to more formal opportunities such as professional programmes or journal clubs. Although some of these activities may be considered informal, you still need clear reasons for pursuing them and the outcomes still need to be measured.

Why would you undertake work-based learning?

Work-based learning is a good way of transferring knowledge by bridging the 'theory to practice' gap and ensuring that practice is immediately enhanced by this new knowledge. As work-based learning activities are usually provided on an in-house basis, they are cost-effective (Lloyd, Pfeiffer et al. 2014) and provide an excellent way for staff in the organisation to share their skills and experience while developing their own skills further. For example, shadowing a colleague can help to broaden your own practice skills while also enabling you to share your knowledge in this area with your colleague.

How would you measure the success of your work-based learning?

As the aim of work-based learning is to improve outcomes for service users, staff and the organisation, its success needs to be measured by analysing changes in these areas. For example, if you have been working to develop your clinical skills in one specific area, has your intervention had a positive impact for your service users in terms of performance, speed of recovery or length of stay? It is sometimes difficult to measure this impact accurately without a purposely designed research project. However, you may only require presentation of case studies and/or positive feedback from your supervisor, colleagues, service users and/or carers, as evidence to satisfy re-registration requirements. You may subsequently decide that a specifically designed research project is required (see 'Formal activities' above).

How does work-based learning contribute to your CPD?

As illustrated above, and as with all CPD activities, it is how you apply what you have learnt in order to improve your practice and service delivery, and how this benefits yourself and others (see Chapter 8), that provides you with evidence of your learning to meet the HCPC standards (HCPC 2017a). For further information about work-based learning, see Alsop (2013).

Journal clubs

Journal clubs can be profession-specific or interprofessional and can be used to discuss the evidence surrounding a wide range of subjects. They usually involve a group of people coming together to discuss the merits and limitations of a particular journal article. Alternatively, each person presents evidence from a range of articles on a specific subject. It is also possible to participate in free online journal clubs (see the section on social media in Chapter 7). There is no single way to run a journal club but there are a few important points to bear in mind, whichever format is chosen:

- You should agree on the ground rules and guidelines before the first meeting to ensure that all participants understand their responsibilities in terms of what they should read or search for and the time allowed.
- All evidence presented should be critiqued, preferably using a critique tool such as CASP (Critical Appraisal Skills Programme 2019).

Why should you join a journal club?

Journal clubs are an excellent way to work with others to establish an evidence base to support your practice (Waite & Keenan 2010). This can be invaluable if you are required to demonstrate that you are using the most up-to-date evidence to support your work.

How can you measure the benefit of journal clubs?

- Complete a reading record, including references and a short summary of your findings, to provide evidence that you have undertaken the reading.
- Write or record a reflection to show how you will apply what you have learnt (see Chapter 8).
- Complete an intervention evidence log (see Chapter 8).
- Disseminate what you have learnt to your colleagues or other professionals to demonstrate your understanding, giving consideration to the most effective way to do this (see Chapter 6).
- Assess your level of confidence about your literature searching and critical appraisal skills.

How does being a member of a journal club contribute to your CPD?
- It develops your knowledge of the evidence base.
- It develops your critiquing skills.
- It can help you formulate guidelines for practice to support an intervention.

Professional or external activities
In this context, professional or external activities can be any of the following:
- Activities that relate specifically to your own profession, such as being a placement educator or an active member of a special interest group, or undertaking work for your professional body
- External activities that require you to be working in your professional capacity, such as external examining, activities for a regulatory body (e.g. HCPC re-approvals) or membership of a university or health/social care related committee, or acting as an expert witness
- Specific roles where you have to be a qualified professional in a specific field; you may or may not be required to undertake additional focused training (e.g. to become an approved mental health practitioner or non-medical prescriber)
- External activities where your professional qualification is not necessarily a prerequisite but the learning obtained contributes to your overall professional practice (e.g. volunteering for a charity or third sector organisation, or undertaking public service duties).

Why would you undertake professional/external activities?
Professional/external activities are excellent career development opportunities, as they can provide you with an overview of the organisation/s for which you are working/acting in an advisory capacity. They can also help to broaden your knowledge in various areas that can be applied to influence your professional practice. Even within a special interest group (although the focus is usually on a specialist area), rich learning opportunities can be provided in relation to specialist practice across a wide range of locations or professions.

How would you measure the success of your professional/external activities?
The success of your professional/external activities can be measured in a variety of ways, especially if it is regularly cross-referenced back to your original learning objectives. If you have undertaken specific training, a certificate or qualification may be a useful measurement of success in relation to your professional activities. However, other specific measurements need to be designed around the individual activity. For example, you may set your own individual targets; or, if you are an external examiner, success could be measured through positive feedback from the institution regarding your contribution and responses to your suggestions.

How do professional/external activities contribute to your CPD?
- They lead to improved formal report-writing skills.
- They can sometimes provide specific management or leadership skills.
- They provide essential networks to support professional practice, such as active participation in Heads of Service meetings.
- They give you greater political and contextual awareness, which can enhance your professional practice.
- They increase your awareness of new developments in knowledge, practice and technology.
- They help you develop advanced professional and interprofessional communication skills.
- They enhance your employability and potentially help to improve your career prospects.

Professional support

Professional support refers to the types of roles and responsibilities undertaken at your place of work. These can include:

- Supervision – a structured process implemented within the workplace to increase understanding of practice and management issues, reflect on their impact on practice and the service user and to drive evidence-based and high-quality practice. Many strategies are in place to support supervision. Although supervision as an activity does not necessarily constitute CPD, the outcomes of your formal discussions may form part of your personal and professional development.
- Mentorship – this can be either formal or informal and is designed to support the long-term professional development of an individual or group. The focus is on the facilitation of learning through a supportive environment, rather than overseeing and guiding practice (as in supervision).
- Coaching – usually provided by an external facilitator. Coaching enables people to identify their learning needs in relation to their role or future aspirations. It also provides strategies to enable them to analyse and achieve their learning objectives.
- Preceptorship (or equivalent) – a process for newly qualified practitioners to guide, facilitate and measure development of professional skills during the formative stages of their careers (HEE 2019). There are also various profession and work context specific learning and development frameworks available (see Chapter 3, Table 3.1).

These roles may or may not be undertaken with people from your own profession. (See also Chapter 9 for more in-depth information on the above professional support activities.)

Why would you undertake professional support?

In the health sector, supervision is a requirement of clinical governance, and preceptorship was introduced as a requirement within Agenda for Change. Similar approaches to professional support are in use across health and social care. Although mentorship and coaching are not mandatory, all these activities have similar benefits, which are to promote professional practice and therefore increase provision of high-quality care for all service users.

How would you measure the success of professional support?

- Through its impact on job satisfaction, confidence and competence in the role, and through staff retention
- Through positive feedback from service users
- Through confirmed achievement of objectives set through supervision, appraisal and
- professional development review processes.

How does professional support contribute to your CPD?

All the above activities facilitate CPD but, in order to count as CPD, it is important that you – as an individual – fully engage with each process. On their own, they have little or no impact on your professional development.

These activities can help you:

- Develop greater confidence and ability in your professional role
- Develop your understanding of professional issues and their application
- Gain opportunities to develop skills in reflection
- Find a forum for the sharing of good practice
- Access opportunities to consider and test out strategies to improve practice
- Develop your ability to work with others by making links between knowledge and personal experience.

Training

Training consists of CPD activities such as courses, attending and/or presenting at conferences (see Chapter 6) and workshops or facilitating/chairing these events. These are usually short scheduled activities, for which you may need to formally apply. You may also need to seek permission from your manager for funding and/or time to attend. They are often themed events, with presenters who are considered experts in their fields – for example, your professional body peer-reviewed annual conference, specialist skill or assessment training or a specific CPD workshop. Training can also include courses that provide accreditation for taking students on practice or clinical placements. These events are often advertised as 'meeting CPD requirements' or 'CPD accredited' (for instance, courses where a CPD certificate is awarded for attending and/or points may be attached).

Although mandatory training should be recorded, it does not usually count as CPD activity in itself, as it is compulsory training to ensure safe practice, rather than training selected to advance your professional development. It is, however, possible to learn something in mandatory training that you later apply in practice to benefit yourself, your service users and/or others (see Chapter 8).

Why would you undertake training?

You might decide to undertake training because you have:

- Identified a learning need with your manager during a supervision or annual review
- Identified a learning need independently – for your career development or in an area of work you would like to move into, or because you know your organisation is keen to promote and engage with an area of practice.

Most people will opt to attend formal training because they wish to update themselves on current developments – for example, the latest evidence to support their practice across their profession from within the UK and further afield. They may also wish to develop their knowledge and skills in a specialist area of practice, where there is no expertise within their organisation.

Formal training events enable you to build links and professional networks outside your organisation; they also offer opportunities to promote your own best practice and research. Some people attend these events to restore their faith in their profession and to re-motivate themselves. Others may never have attended a formal event but have perhaps been inspired to attend by colleagues. Some have attended but feel they have not benefited; this may be because they have not prepared thoroughly or have not made the most of opportunities that were available (see Chapter 1, case study).

In order to attend a formal training event, you may need to negotiate funding with your manager. If this is the case, it is important to ensure that you have explicitly identified a learning need in your annual review, appraisal or supervision (see Chapters 9 and 10). Once you have identified an appropriate formal training opportunity, you need to thoroughly investigate the details of the programme, presenters and full potential costs – including travel, accommodation, subsistence and fees.

You can present your evidence of identified learning needs, using TRAMmCPD, through supervision or review/appraisal. You will need to:

- Clearly demonstrate why and how your chosen formal training event will meet your objectives
- Refer to any evidence that is available to support the need for your attendance – for example, a new treatment where there is currently no internal skill base
- Look at professional body websites where there may be templates available for letters to apply for funding and/or present a business case for why you should be allowed to attend
- Demonstrate how your attendance will benefit your organisation and how you will disseminate the information on your return (see Chapter 6)

- Consider alternative funding sources so that your employer may only need to give you study leave (for instance, your professional body, charities, academies, companies, part self-funding).

How do you measure the effectiveness of formal training?

The effectiveness of formal training can be measured in many and varied ways, depending upon the nature and purpose of the event. (For details, see Chapter 10.)

How to get the most out of conferences

Before the conference

- Obtain a copy of the conference programme at the earliest opportunity, ideally before the event itself so that you have time to study it in depth; programmes can initially appear very complicated so ask someone who has attended previously for their assistance.
- Identify and highlight the most appropriate events in the conference programme, making notes about their location within the venue, particularly if you will need to move swiftly between sessions.

During the conference:

- If you use social media and decide to communicate during sessions, study the conference social media guidelines, and ensure you adhere to your professional code of conduct. Use the agreed conference code or hashtag (e.g. Twitter #).
- Download any conference tools, such as apps, online timetables or abstracts.
- To make the best use of your time, identify your priorities, check for clashes and ensure you have booked your place in any sessions where this is required.
- Allow time to view posters and exhibitors' stands.
- Make time to network with others – you will be surprised how much you can gain from this.
- Make notes, doodles and reflections, as you think of them.

After the conference

- Complete your running CPD record (e.g. TRAMm Tracker, see Chapter 7) with brief details of your attendance.
- Write more detailed notes (e.g. initiate a TRAMm Trail, see Chapter 7) with details of the sessions you attended, what you learnt and how you will use the information and contacts to benefit your organisation and service users.
- Follow up with any contacts made during the conference (for instance, send an email, connect on social media, telephone call)
- Consider how you will disseminate what you have learnt to your colleagues and manager (see Chapter 6).

- Think about how you will apply what you learnt at the conference to benefit your service users (see Chapter 8).
- At your next supervision, discuss using the TRAMm Tracker and TRAMm Trail to summarise the benefits of your attendance and your future plans.

How does this type of training contribute to your CPD?

Training provided through courses, workshops and conferences is one of the most commonly considered activities for CPD because people believe that these activities can provide quick, easily accessible evidence, with supporting CPD certificates or credit points.

In order to meet the HCPC standards (HCPC 2017a), it is essential to include evidence showing how the training has affected your practice and improved outcomes for service users and others. This should be the focus of your subsequent reflections and your plans for your future learning needs, which can be recorded.

How to get the most out of courses and workshops

The principles are similar to those that apply when attending a conference (see above) but there may be some differences.

Before the course or workshop

- Complete any required pre-course reading or work (e.g. pre-course e-module)
- Undertake background reading if no prerequisite work or prior knowledge of the subject has been specified
- Consider your own expectations and objectives for attending to ensure that these are addressed
- Check whether there are any clothing or other special requirements for the day
- Find out whether lunch and refreshments are provided.

After the course or workshop

- Complete your running CPD record (e.g. TRAMm Tracker, see Chapter 7), including the title of the training event and the date.
- For the most significant sessions, initiate a TRAMm Trail (see Chapter 7), including what you attended, what you learnt and how you will use the information and contacts to benefit your organisation, service users and others.
- Consider how you will disseminate what you learnt to your colleagues and manager (see Chapter 6).
- Think about how you will apply what you have learnt to benefit your service users (see Chapter 8).

- At your next supervision, discuss using the TRAMm Tracker and TRAMm Trail to summarise the benefits of your attendance and your future plans.

Informal support

CPD often starts with an activity, and informal support can be the first in a series of CPD activities relating to a specific area of skill or knowledge development. Informal support does not always begin as an explicit CPD activity; instead you may find yourself in a situation where you suddenly recognise there are learning opportunities at your disposal.

Informal support can be received or provided in a number of ways and can include, for example, peer group support, informal mentorship, and ad hoc discussion forums (such as discussions in the staff room or office). Journal clubs may also fit in this category if they are locally organised within a department, although they can also be arranged more formally if they are part of larger interprofessional events.

Informal support may advance your learning or provide the impetus for further learning to occur. An example might be a scenario in a staff room, where a colleague informally shares her experience of a recent course where she learnt about a new intervention. You may discuss how the intervention can be useful with your specific service user group, or it may provide an incentive to find out more and attend a course yourself. Either way, you may be developing your professional knowledge and understanding of a specific area.

Why would you undertake informal support?

Informal support can usually be accessed more quickly than formal support and is often more timely for you and your service user/s. However, it is important to be clear on how these informal activities contribute to your CPD, rather than just being 'normal' work activities. For example, in the above scenario in the staff room, if you listen to your colleague and ask a few questions about what she is discussing with others, this can just be considered a normal workplace activity involving sharing of information. However, if you use this discussion as a springboard to further your interest and then undertake some research, take your ideas to supervision and undertake other related learning activities in order to apply what you have learnt to your service user group, this may contribute considerably to your CPD. This process can be usefully reflected and recorded on a TRAMm Trail.

How would you measure the success of informal support?

It is often more difficult to measure the success of informal support, although it can be linked to service user outcomes if it is a very clear and specific activity (see Chapter 10 for more information on measuring your CPD).

How does informal support contribute to your CPD?

Informal support does not, in and of itself, count as CPD but, depending on the informal support received or provided, it can contribute to CPD in various ways. It is therefore important to remind

yourself of the HCPC definition and standards required of CPD (as outlined in Chapter 1) in order to recognise CPD opportunities as they are presented. Informal support may:
- Form part of a series of activities designed to further your knowledge and skills
- Initiate or inform reflection on a specific situation or service user.

Social media

Social media uses online technology to enable and encourage social interactions. It has become increasingly popular as the quickest and most cost-effective way to keep up to date with legislation, guidelines and research. Using social media can be an effective method of networking with like-minded people, including professionals, people with lived experience and service users, both locally and internationally. Social media can also be used to promote your skills or service and disseminate or discuss good practice.

There are many different types of social media, including apps, blogs, information collation tools, video sharing, online communities, document sharing, and social and business networking sites. Discussion forums, online chats and online journal clubs are becoming increasingly popular ways of using social networking sites to participate in CPD. These can help to encourage intraprofessional and interprofessional communication via profession-specific and CPD-specific groups on popular social networking sites. Here you can pose questions to the wider community, follow conference sessions and make comments. These suggestions are by no means exhaustive; as technology advances, the methods and sites available are constantly changing and evolving.

Whichever type of online networking you use, it is important to adhere to the social media guidelines provided by the HCPC (HCPC 2017b), your professional body and organisation/employer. It is also imperative that you are fully aware of your professional code of ethics and conduct, as this applies to all your online interactions across all platforms, whether professional or social. It is *always* vital to maintain service user/colleague confidentiality, in all interactions. Links to (or hard copies of) your social media interactions or collations may contribute to your CPD, if they help provide evidence of how you have met the HCPC standards for CPD, rather than just being an activity you enjoy. (See Chapter 8 for further discussion of things you need to consider before you apply your learning from your use of social media.)

Why would you use social media?

There are many reasons why you might wish to engage with aspects of social media, including:
- It is free to use and cost-effective – there is no charge to use most sites, and no printing or postal costs
- It provides networking opportunities and allows the promotion of research, products organisations and professional body activities

- It can provide professional support if you work in an isolated area, feel isolated, or you are receiving supervision from a different profession
- It can enhance communication and allow you to engage with a wider audience, which can include professionals, commissioners, service users and carers
- Responses can be instant so you can obtain swift answers to queries or ideas from others that you had not considered
- It can broaden your perspective.

Despite all these benefits, it is important to remember that, to some, the vast array of social media activities available can appear daunting and overwhelming. There can be a fear of open criticism and abuse and a concern about getting things wrong, especially as interactions are viewed by so many people.

If you are a novice user of social media and would like to get involved, talk to colleagues to see what they are using and stick to your own professional sites. You do not always have to participate; you can 'lurk' to observe what is going on and to gain an understanding of how people interact.

For suggestions about how to use social media to develop your own learning communities, see Chapter 6. Chapter 7 includes ideas about how to record your learning from your social media use and Chapter 8 contains suggestions for things you need to consider before you apply your learning from your social media use.

How can you capture your social media use?

- Complete your running CPD record (e.g. TRAMm Tracker, see Chapter 7) including dates with relevant links.
- For your most significant sessions and interactions, include additional details, e.g. initiate a TRAMm Trail – include what you contributed to, and where to access the information in the future
- Download transcripts or take and save screenshots of significant interactions
- Develop an understanding of, and use, different media to save or record useful information, e.g. digital collation and curation (see Chapter 7)
- Keep a record of how you plan to use what you have learnt to benefit your practice, organisation, service users and others.
- Consider how you can disseminate what you have learnt to your colleagues and/or manager and the best way to do this
- Write or record a reflection to show how you will apply what you have learnt.

How does social media interaction contribute to CPD?

- It can help you build wider professional networks and broaden your perspective.
- It can provide immediate, up-to-date knowledge of new developments.

- It can enable participation in activities, such as online journal clubs, to critically evaluate evidence and aspects of practice.
- It can help you develop your skills of critical analysis and judge the credibility of information (see Chapter 8).
- It can provide a forum to discuss and debate current issues related to practice and to consider your own position in relation to these, which may encourage you to make positive changes to your practice
- It can also contribute to your running record of evidence of participation in CPD activities.

How can you measure the success of your use of social media?

This very much depends on the context of your learning, what you have learnt and how you have used and applied your learning in practice to benefit yourself and others (see Chapter 8). For example, as a researcher, you may need to consider impact factors and the analytics of your social media interactions. As a practitioner, you may need to consider the impact your social media use has on your learning, how it has influenced your practice and its impact on yourself, your team, the people who access your service, your organisation and/or wider stakeholders. Chapter 10 discusses how to measure your learning from a range of CPD-related activities.

Self-directed learning

Self-directed learning is anything that is undertaken on an individual and informal basis that helps to expand learning or knowledge. This can involve activities such as e-learning, including the use of multimedia technology for learning and informal research, reading journal articles and speaking to other professionals and agencies. According to Knowles (1975, p. 18):

> 'In its broadest meaning, 'self-directed learning' describes a process by which individuals take the initiative, with or without the assistance of others, in diagnosing their learning needs, formulating learning goals, identifying human and material resources for learning, choosing and implementing appropriate learning strategies, and evaluating learning outcomes.'

Self-directed learning can help to increase confidence, self-efficacy and motivation (Boyer, Edmondson, et al. 2013). (For more details, see Chapter 4.)

Why would you undertake self-directed learning?

Self-directed learning can be a quick and easy way to establish knowledge, as it relies upon no one else and can usually be easily resourced. Within the introduction to TRAMmCPD (Chapter 5), we establish that CPD is a personal and individual journey. In applying the process of self-directed learning (Knowles 1975), you as the individual would decide what you need to learn, the resources and strategies you need to support this learning, and how you will know if you have been successful.

How would you measure the success of your self-directed learning?
The success of self-directed learning can be measured in a variety of ways but will particularly be cross-referenced back to the original objectives of your learning. For further information about measuring your CPD, see Chapter 10.

How does self-directed learning contribute to your CPD?
- Extended knowledge is carried forward into future working practices.
- It may put you in a position to offer advice to others in similar situations in future.
- It can help you develop useful professional networks for future learning opportunities.
- It gives you an opportunity to gain knowledge of the roles of other professional colleagues.

Reflection
Reflection is a complex process of analysis, critical awareness and self-evaluation that results in a change of practice. Webster-Wright (2009) highlights the central significance of critical reflection in effective professional development. She emphasises that the act of questioning assumptions and taken-for-granted practice can lead to effective professional learning and subsequent change in practice.

Such reflection ideally occurs in the context of the workplace, to enable the most efficient and effective professional learning to take place. Dall'Alba and Sandberg (2006) support this view, encouraging organisations to promote critical reflection in order to facilitate the understanding of practice or 'professional ways of being' (p. 402) which lead to skill development. They suggest that this reflection can be encouraged through focused dialogue in the context where the issue arises – in health and care professions this would usually be the clinical setting.

Reflection is more effectively undertaken verbally, or via a written record, following a structured model. This approach facilitates consideration of all the issues surrounding the topic, including those that may be challenging personal values and beliefs and their impact on what you are trying to achieve (see Chapter 7).

Reflection can be undertaken as an internal conversation on an informal and regular basis. Alternatively, more formal verbal and written reflections can be used to address areas where greater understanding and awareness are required. Models and methods of reflection are covered in more depth in Chapter 7; and Moon (2004) contains some useful resources to enable you to reflect effectively.

Why would you undertake reflection?
Reflection is undertaken to allow practitioners to attempt to make sense of what they have done or to consider outcomes and critical events. The main aim is to help consolidate learning and develop practice.

How would you measure the success of your reflections?
- Reflection enables you to clearly document and express antecedents, behaviours and consequences contributing to an event or situation.

- Your reflection shows that you have made a positive change to your practice, which impacts on your service users, team and/or organisation; success can then be measured through feedback, observation or outcome measure.
- If you initiate a TRAMm Tracker event, you can record the fact that reflection has been undertaken.
- You can also measure its success according to how clearly you can disseminate what you have learnt to others.

How does reflection contribute to your CPD?

- Reflective models provide a vehicle through which you can consider and adapt your professional practice.
- Written reflections can also provide evidence of your clinical reasoning and how you have used newly gained knowledge and skills to influence your practice and benefit service users and others.
- Reflection can help you identify future learning needs
- Reflection can also occur when working in emerging or non-traditional roles or taking a career break.

This chapter has only illustrated a few of the most common forms of CPD activity to show the possible range, but there are a great many other activities that could be included. If you are in a non-traditional, emerging role or are taking a career break, you need to be a little more creative in how you match your CPD activities to the HCPC standards for proficiency and CPD (HCPC 2017a). For most this is possible, although the complexity of this creative challenge varies depending on your particular professional group.

Emerging or non-traditional roles are those where you may be using some or all of your professional skills but not necessarily explicitly (Treseder 2012) – for example, working as a care home manager or in a women's refuge. You could be on a career break but working part-time as a sports coach, running a playgroup or working in a café. In each of these cases, it is important to consider the demands of the role and how the skills you are using or developing link to those required for your profession. For example, if you are running a playgroup you could be developing your skills of leadership, communicating with children or learning about the value of play. In contrast, if you are in a women's refuge, you may be learning more about working with people who have suffered significant psychological or physical abuse or about managing conflict.

To maintain or renew your registration in such circumstances, you will still need to consider how to evidence your CPD. It is important to find an approach that suits you, decide how and what you will measure, and seek the support of a mentor from your profession to act as a sounding board and give you guidance (see Chapter 9). Remember that it is always possible to keep learning and developing, do not give up purely because you are no longer working in an explicitly professional role.

Case study: Sally undertakes a mixture of activities

In the first chapter we introduced Sally, an occupational therapist who was funded by her employer to attend a two-day conference, where she went to several ad hoc sessions with no forethought or planning.

In a staff meeting a colleague who has been on a TRAMmCPD workshop gives a brief overview of the HCPC standards for CPD and how TRAMmCPD can help to ensure engagement in CPD. It is important to engage in a range of learning activities to do CPD and Sally realises that she has only attended one conference and that is not enough to meet the HCPC standards. Following a team discussion, the team agree that a journal club will be arranged once a month, for one hour, over lunch. The first article selected for review is Hearle and Lawson (2019) on CPD engagement, as it is relevant for all staff.

- How many different types of learning activities is Sally now doing?
- What else could Sally do to make the most of her learning?
- Which HCPC standards of CPD is Sally meeting at this point?
- What other activities could Sally engage in to learn and develop?

Tasks

The following tasks will encourage you to consider the activities you have already undertaken and reflect on the most significant. This will enable you to consider your identified learning needs and intended outcomes.

1. Consider two of the most recent and significant learning activities you have undertaken (one formal, one informal) and use a reflective model (see Chapter 7) to articulate why they have been significant, what you have learned, and what you intend to change or develop in your practice as a result.

2. Think about the types of activities you currently undertake. Can you identify other types of activity you could engage in to widen the scope of your CPD? Remember to be realistic in terms of cost, time and other resources available.

3. If you are a newly qualified member of staff, or returning to practice, check with your professional body for preceptorship and/or career/learning and development frameworks to support your practice.

4. Think about the activities you are already undertaking that could be considered as CPD or could easily be developed further to become CPD. It may be useful to discuss this with colleagues. This exercise will be especially helpful if you are working in extended scope/emerging roles or are currently taking a career break.

5. Consider how you might use one of these activities to demonstrate that you have met HCPC CPD standards 1–4 (HCPC 2017a).

6. Read Chapter 3 to discover how to adopt a more creative approach to your CPD.

3

Taking responsibility for CPD: Changing mindsets

This chapter aims to inspire you to adopt a creative approach to CPD. Whilst reading, you will be encouraged to consider and reflect upon your own responsibilities in relation to your personal and professional development, as well as the rewards of adopting a proactive approach to CPD engagement.

This chapter will also explore the recommended responsibilities for employers and wider networks and how they can help support you in this area. In addition, it will discuss how to design internal structures, recognise everyday learning and access formal CPD without funds, with suggestions for building a case to attend formal training.

Tasks at the end of the chapter will encourage you to consider and document your CPD plans, with suggestions for how your employers/networks might provide support. You will also be encouraged to consider structures within your team or organisation which could enable CPD. We have also included a template showing you how to build a case to attend formal training that can be adapted if you wish to develop your own.

Why do you need to think differently?

At a recent conference, a healthcare professional presenting a full-service evaluation they had undertaken in their workplace, was overheard stating 'it's great to be here at this conference as I haven't done any CPD for several years'. What is wrong with this statement?

Despite all that is written on CPD, and clear guidance from the HCPC (2017a) and other health and care professional bodies about the need to value a range of learning activities as counting towards CPD, perceptions like this are not uncommon. In the above scenario, the service evaluation itself clearly provided an excellent professional development opportunity – and later in this chapter we will explain why.

Professionals frequently point to the lack of resources in the health and social care sectors as factors preventing CPD from taking place (Lawson 2018, Hearle & Lawson 2019, Lawson & Tempest 2019). However, in organisations where financial limitations will always be an issue, we must begin to think differently about what constitutes CPD. Rather than think of ways to 'undertake' formal CPD, we should instead consider what we are already doing, or can do, to contribute to our personal development. We hear a lot in practice about the need to 'work smarter and more effectively' and this can also be applied to our own CPD.

So, how do we change our mindset about how we view, recognise and articulate what contributes to our CPD? The remainder of this chapter will explore the responsibilities we all have, in terms of professional development, and the benefits of upholding these responsibilities. It will also provide some practical examples of how we can change our mindsets to enable us to engage in CPD more easily.

What are your responsibilities in relation to your personal and professional development?

Knowles (1975) described self-directed learning (SDL) as a process in which the learner is responsible for managing their own learning throughout a learning activity and this approach can clearly be applied to CPD. Empirical research has demonstrated that SDL can foster a number of positive factors, including enhanced academic performance, aspiration, creativity, curiosity and life satisfaction (Edmondson, Boyer & Artis 2012, Boyer, Edmondson, et al. (2013).

Recognising the potential in every opportunity is central to your responsibility as a professional. In their joint principles for health and social care professionals, Broughton and Harris (2019) stress the importance of recognising and demonstrating the effects of CPD and lifelong learning on practice. In addition, they emphasise the importance of recognising the value of both planned and unplanned learning. Dall'Alba (2009, p. 34) states:

> 'Learning to become a professional involves not only what we know and can do, but also who we are (becoming). It involves integration of knowing, acting, and being in the form of professional ways of being that unfold over time...while knowledge and skills are necessary, they are insufficient for skilful practice and for transformation of the self that is integral to achieving such practice.'

Dall'Alba is referring here to the professional development of students. However, this theory could also apply to CPD for practitioners. The fact that students and practitioners can learn the same information and be able to carry out the same activities, while still appearing to have completely different levels of skill and expertise, suggests that there is more to professional learning and development than simply the acquisition of skills and knowledge.

In an earlier paper, Dall'Alba and Sandberg (2006) discuss the importance of a person's perception and understanding of their own practice, alongside their knowledge and skills. They discuss the limitations of the container model in relation to teaching where curricula evidence the belief that skills and theory can be taught separately and will automatically be understood and implemented by the learner when required. They refute the idea of practice as a fixed entity and instead support a more dynamic model where learning depends on the experience of the learner, the context in which they are learning and the translation of learning into practice. This is supported by empirical research (Billett 2001; Borko, Mayfield, et al. 1997; Mol 2002; Webster-Wright 2009). For example, for someone new to an area, it may be useful to understand the underpinning theory before attempting to put it into practice. Likewise, someone who has expertise in a specific area may already understand the theory but this does not mean that they stop learning; they can be encouraged to critique the theory in order to further develop their practice.

This theory can also be seen to play out in the field of health and social care where the varied practices may conflict. An example in occupational therapy may be a case where a person is unable to get into the bath. One occupational therapist may suggest a strip wash or a shower, assuming the core goal for the person as a self-care activity – keeping clean. Another occupational therapist may explore the nature of bathing in terms of the person's occupations. Through this exploration, it may be revealed that bathing is more of a leisure occupation (which enables the individual to relax and refocus at the end of a busy day) or it may contribute to pain relief if the person has a musculoskeletal problem. In the latter case, a strip wash or shower will not suffice, and an alternative solution needs to be identified.

Although both these scenarios relate to what could be considered normal everyday practice, undertaking a reflection may contribute to greater understanding of the situation and help the practitioner develop insight into the factors that influence a person's choice of occupations. Some may consider such a reflection to be CPD. Webster-Wright (2009, p. 715) uses the term 'authentic professional learning' to describe what she states is 'the lived experience of continuing to learn as a professional' and this may be an example of such a lived experience. Continuing professional development can arise from many instances, including day-to-day practice such as the above example. How you might decide when usual everyday work has the potential to become CPD is considered later in this chapter.

In order to fully understand our responsibilities, it is also important to consider the drivers and impact of CPD. Within the UK health and care context, we clearly have mandatory responsibilities which act as important drivers for CPD, such as the requirements of the HCPC and the NMC for nurses and midwives. Whilst we cannot ignore the influence of regulatory body expectations, research also reveals the significance of intrinsic factors in driving our professional development.

Ryan (2003) explores the factors that influence motivation to undertake CPD in three groups of healthcare professionals: nurses, occupational therapists and physiotherapists. Responses on a questionnaire revealed that most of their motivating/driving factors were intrinsic rather than extrinsic. For instance, the desire to update professional knowledge so as not to become 'stale' was a major motivation, alongside a need to update their qualifications, demonstrate their competence and help to raise the profile of their profession.

Penman (2014) also discusses the importance of intrinsic drivers, suggesting that individuals need to be in a position of readiness to learn in order to embrace CPD. It may be useful at this point to consider your own position in relation to this. If you are not 'ready to learn' or motivated in the context you find yourself in, you may wish to consider why this might be the case. In some cases, if the issues are unresolvable, you may need to consider moving to another setting, changing your role or changing direction completely in order to gain a sense of professional fulfilment and be able to practise to the best of your ability.

A study by Gunn and Goding (2009) explored the drivers, engagement and impact of CPD within the physiotherapy profession. A range of drivers for CPD were highlighted by participants, including their identity as professionals and their desire to provide the most effective service to clients. Despite these factors, participants revealed that their actual engagement with CPD activities (such as reflection and portfolio keeping) was limited, and attributed this to a lack of skills in these areas. These learning needs could be addressed informally within teams or via mentorship and do not necessarily need courses or formal training.

There are clear links between engaging in CPD and job satisfaction and this is important for both employees and employers. For employees, there is strong evidence to show that those who actively engage in CPD experience greater satisfaction in their role and are more likely to be respected and progress in their career more quickly (Van den Broeck, Vansteenkiste, et al. 2008, Schaufeli & Bakker 2004). For employers, there is also evidence linking contented practitioners, who are supported to engage in CPD, with staff retention and avoidance of burnout. When there is significant investment in CPD (whether individually or via organisational policy), the individual feels valued and is happy in their work and their quality of practice is shown to improve (Van den Broeck, Vansteenkiste, et al. 2008, Schaufeli & Bakker 2004, NHS Staff Council 2009). In contrast, when CPD is given limited attention or people are disengaged at work, this has been shown to correlate with work-related stress and burnout, resulting in increased staff sickness, absence and subsequent decreased productivity (Van den Broeck, Vansteenkiste, et al. 2008, Schaufeli & Bakker 2004, Poulsen, Meredith, et al. 2014).

This brief review suggests that it can be mutually beneficial for individuals who are motivated to engage in CPD to work in a culture that values CPD and encourages them to actively engage in it. Broughton and Harris (2019) emphasise that the individual should take responsibility for their own learning, but that line managers and organisations also have a responsibility to develop a culture where learning and advancement of practice is valued and positively supported.

How do you know when your learning has the potential to become CPD?

In order to change your thinking about CPD, it is important to have something to guide your thinking and enable you to make these decisions. There are frameworks which can help with this, including the defining attributes for CPD engagement (Hearle & Lawson 2019) and Desimone's four-stage framework (Desimone 2009).

The stages of successful professional development

Desimone (2009, p. 184), suggests that it is possible to provide a four-stage framework for successful professional development which will help to measure the success of the professional development process. Although she initially constructed these in relation to teaching, it is possible to apply these stages to healthcare, as shown in Figure 3.1.

---

1. You have learnt something new

   ↓

2. Your learning increases your knowledge and skills, and changes your attitudes and/or values

   ↓

3. You use your new knowledge and skills to improve your practice

   ↓

4. This change in practice should improve the quality of your practice and patient outcomes.

Figure 3.1 Stages of successful professional development (adapted from Desimone 2009, p.184)

It can be useful to examine yourself against these stages to determine whether you have indeed been undertaking CPD. Once you have done this, Desimone argues it is then possible to assess the effectiveness of your professional development by answering three questions:

1. Do you learn?
2. Do you change your practice?
3. Do patient outcomes improve?

Desimone's ideas certainly provide a useful framework. However, service user outcomes may be harder to measure as it is difficult to attribute them solely to the development of the professional.

Taking this framework further, it is useful to consider the concept of CPD engagement which is explored in the following section.

Engaging in CPD

Much of the literature pertaining to CPD, including regulations and guidance documents for most health and care professionals (HCPC 2017a, Broughton & Harris 2019), highlights the need for individuals to engage in CPD. However, in many instances the meaning of the term 'engagement' is unclear. A concept analysis, conducted in preparation for a research project into the effectiveness of the TRAMm Model (Hearle & Lawson 2019), identified the following defining attributes of CPD engagement:

1. CPD is self-initiated and undertaken voluntarily, rather than as a result of a mandatory requirement.
2. The individual feels rewarded, either intrinsically (e.g. enjoyment) or extrinsically (e.g. promotion), during or after undertaking CPD.
3. The knowledge/skills gained through the CPD are embraced and applied in practice for the benefit of the service/service user.
4. Learning is recorded, evaluated and/or shared with others
5. Learning is shown to continue beyond the initial CPD activity.

In order to fully understand the meaning and application of these attributes, it may help to analyse the following constructed case examples 3.1–3.4 (Hearle & Lawson 2019, pp. 254–256). Example 3.1 illustrates CPD engagement in its entirety, if using the defining attributes above. If you think you are doing something similar to this, you can assume that you are fully engaging in your professional development. If you are unsure, it may be helpful to try to separate the defining attributes in Example 3.1 and then apply this to your own situation. If you find that you relate more to one of the other cases (Examples 3.2–3.4), highlighting the areas you may be missing might enable you to recognise learning as it is happening.

Example 3.1 CPD engagement model case

This is an example reflecting all five of the defining attributes of CPD engagement:

Jess is a Band 7 Occupational Therapist who leads the Occupational Therapy team on a Stroke Unit. She was delighted this month to read an article in the *British Journal of Occupational Therapists* about Constraint Induced Movement Therapy as a new technique encouraging a return to function for people who had suffered a stroke. She uses the internet to explore further evidence of this approach and contacts the authors (an occupational therapist and physiotherapist) who agree that she can spend a few days with them, observing and learning how to apply the approach in practice.

Jess prepares a case to negotiate the time from work in supervision. Following her experience, she makes detailed notes and reflects on her experience. On her return to work, she selects four patients on which to trial the new approach, taking a baseline measurement of ability before she begins the treatment and re-measuring four weeks later.

Excited by the results, she writes a report for the clinical director and prepares an in-service training session for the whole team, with a more detailed hands-on training for the local occupational therapy special interest group. She documents her activity on a TRAMm Tracker and provides more detail on a TRAMm Trail, which she files in her portfolio alongside her reflection and report, as she knows this will provide useful evidence if she is called for audit by the HCPC.

Example 3.2 CPD engagement contrary case

This is an example reflecting none of the defining attributes of CPD engagement:

Joe, a Band 6 Physiotherapist, considers supervision a waste of time but attends as it is compulsory within his workplace. His line manager reminds him that he has not undertaken any CPD over the last 18 months and as a HCPC registered professional it is his responsibility.

To 'keep his supervisor off his back', he finds a one-day free course on something to do with a new piece of legislation, which some of his colleagues are going to. During the course he listens to the introduction and then gets bored. He spends the rest of the day making a list of all the things he needs to sort for his holiday in a few weeks' time and investigates the best surfing beaches on his tablet. At the end of the day he collects his certificate and puts it in his drawer to show to his supervisor the next time they meet.

Example 3.3 CPD engagement related case

This case has many but not all the defining attributes of CPD engagement:

Sue is a Band 8a Nurse who wishes to move from her current post on an acute medical ward, where she has been for the last five years, to a new role in education. She is coming to the end of her Masters degree which she commenced because she knew it would help her secure a post in the University sector. With the support of her organisation (in terms of time off and full funding), Sue has enjoyed studying again and is proud that her average grades have reached 65% and above. She has been a student mentor within the workplace and has developed new student mentorship strategies following a project she undertook during her recent studies. Until recently, Sue was undertaking some sessional teaching, although this has stopped since she was told by her manager that she had to do it in her own time as she was being paid.

Explanation: This case is related: CPD defining attributes 1, 2 and 3 are either met or partly met, although motivation for being a sessional speaker is questionable since payment stopped. In relation to defining attributes 4 and 5, there is no evidence of recording or evaluating CPD (with the exception of assignments) and learning beyond CPD activity is possible but not explicit.

Example 3.4 CPD engagement borderline case

It is unclear whether or not this example represents CPD engagement:

Jackie is a Band 5 Dietitian who is two years into her first post on a Stroke Unit in a busy teaching hospital. She has undertaken a couple of one-day update courses on nutrition for patients with a PEG feed and undertakes a reflection following each one. She also attends an interprofessional journal club that is held on the unit every two months, where there is a CPD feedback session and presentation prior to the journal discussion.

Next week it is Jackie's turn to present something on the dietitian's role with people who are PEG fed, prior to discussing the article. She is therefore preparing her presentation and has checked the internet to make sure she has the most up-to-date information. She places a copy of this presentation alongside her course reflections in her portfolio.

Explanation: This case appears to meet the defining attributes of CPD engagement. The elements which are unclear are the levels of autonomy, in terms of choice of CPD and degree of application in practice. However, the courses do relate to her work on the unit so choice and application could be assumed. There is also little indication of drive/motivation and reward but again this could be implicit, as she strives to make sure her information is current, which suggests pride in her work.

Defining attribute 2 suggests that you should feel some sense of reward, either intrinsically (e.g. enjoyment) or extrinsically (e.g. promotion), during or after undertaking CPD. In relation to this, it may be useful for you to consider those aspects of your role that are providing you with such rewards. If you feel unable to highlight any rewards derived from your current role, consider aspects that are within your control which may help you to change this.

You may need to take some time to take stock of where you are in your career and look at other possibilities beyond your current situation. To help you do this, there are various frameworks available for health and social care professionals based on the four core Pillars of Practice: Clinical Practice; Facilitation of Learning; Leadership; Evidence, Research and Development (NHS Education for Scotland 2012). These can help you identify ways to challenge your current mindset and move forward in a more positive way to achieve the rewards you are seeking. See Table 3.1 below for some examples of frameworks; there are others available and more in development.

Table 3.1 Examples of learning and development frameworks

Allied Health Professions Critical Care Professional Development Framework (Intensive Care Society 2018) https://www.ics.ac.uk/ICS/Resources___AHP_Framework.aspx (Accessed 26.2.2020)
Allied Health Professions Framework for Wales (Welsh Government 2019)　https://gov.wales/allied-health-professions-ahp-framework (Accessed 26.2.2020)
Learning and Development Framework for Occupational Therapists new or returning to social care (Skills for Care and RCOT 2019) https://www.skillsforcare.org.uk/Learning-development/Regulated-professionals/Occupational-therapists.aspx (Accessed 26.2.2020)

Occupational Therapists in Social Care; a learning and development framework (Social Care Wales and RCOT (2017). https://socialcare.wales/cms_assets/file-uploads/Occupational-therapists-in-social-care_A-learning-and-development-framew.._-002.pdf (Accessed 26.2.2020)
Physiotherapy Framework (Condensed version): putting physiotherapy behaviours, values, knowledge & skills into practice (Chartered Society of Physiotherapy. 2013) https://www.csp.org.uk/system/files/documents/2018-06/csp_physiotherapy_framework_condensed_2013.pdf (Accessed 26.2.2020) (The full framework can be accessed for members via the CSP website.)
Post Registration Career Development Framework Scotland http://www.careerframework.nes.scot.nhs.uk/using-the-framework/pillars-of-practice.aspx (Accessed 26.2.2020)
Principles for CPD and Lifelong Learning in Health and Social Care (Broughton & Harris 2019) https://www.bda.uk.com/training/cpd/cpdjointstatement https://www.csp.org.uk/system/files/documents/2019-01/cpd_principles.pdf (Accessed 3. 4.2020)
The Career Development Framework: Guiding Principles for Occupational Therapy. The Royal College of Occupational Therapists (RCOT 2017) https://www.rcot.co.uk/cpd-rcot. (Accessed 26.2.2020)

It could be that you are ready for a new challenge, in which case the frameworks may help you identify your transferable skills and knowledge alongside those you may need to develop further. Alternatives might be that you look to further develop the role you currently have by reflecting on potential opportunities and thinking creatively about how these might evolve. For example, talking with others who are where you would like to be in your future career or in areas you might be interested in. Ask them how they got there and what they believe helped them to achieve their position. You might also ask your line manager to point you in the direction of the sort of qualifications expected for promotion or movement within or across the four Pillars of Practice. See Chapter 6 (Tell) for more suggestions for ways to find support.

It may be useful to reflect on the CPD activity, to explore the reasons for your lack of engagement or reward. For example, is your lack of reward due to you choosing the wrong type of development activities? Some ideas for models of reflection which might help you are discussed later, along with defining attribute 4).

If you are in practice and struggling to secure funding for traditional CPD activities, try to think creatively about how you might develop your skills effectively without charge. Joining special interest groups is always a good way of sharing skills with like-minded people; you might even meet your next boss!! Or consider making more use of social media. Pursuing areas of interest may provide the reward you need.

Consider what you could measure in terms of a reward. You may have been rewarded without being aware of it. For example, you may be completing tasks more quickly as a result of your CPD or you may have grown in confidence (see Chapter 10).

Defining attribute 3 is that the knowledge and skills gained via the activity are embraced and applied in practice for the benefit of yourself, your service users, the service and your organisation. You might find you are doing this by changing something small in your practice, using a new skill you have learnt, introducing a new system/policy or stopping something you were previously doing that, you now realise, is not evidence based or has been shown to be less effective. If you are doing any of these things, you may be undertaking CPD. Go back to the constructed cases (Examples 3.1–3.4) and try to identify if you are.

Moving to defining attribute 4, the notion that learning needs to be recorded (see Chapter 7), evaluated (see Chapters 9 and 10) and shared with others (see Chapter 6) leads to another question you might ask yourself in order to ascertain if you are undertaking CPD. There are times in your career when you may find yourself being consulted on a subject or asked to teach someone else something that you find easy. It can be a useful exercise to stop and ask yourself, 'how did I get to this point?' This may allow you to identify CPD opportunities you have exploited without knowing. Thinking differently about your CPD and the day-to-day opportunities available to you, it may be useful to look back over things you have recorded within your work over the last couple of weeks and see if there are occasions where you had to look outside your core skill set or turn to others for advice.

How do you know when your normal work practice becomes CPD?

During the pilot evaluation of TRAMmCPD, and following examination of HCPC documentation including their CPD standards (HCPC 2017a), a frequently asked question has been 'How do I know when my routine work activity has developed into CPD?' There is no definitive answer, but considering the following questions may help you answer it:

- Have you reached a point at which you are no longer working on automatic pilot or has something challenged you to stop and think?
- Have you had to look something up or ask others for advice?
- Have you had an emotional reaction that has forced you to reflect? For example, have you felt a sense of frustration, disappointment, discomfort or pride?
- Are you undertaking an activity (see Chapter 2) in order to learn something new?
- Has your usual intervention had an unintended consequence? Have you reflected on the reasons for this and will you change your practice as a result?
- Have you been asked to undertake something new, of which you have little or no experience?
- Have you identified a new way of working through supervision or appraisal, or are you beginning to develop advanced skills in order to further your career?

- Having attended a training event in the past, have you recently used the knowledge gained to improve a service user's outcome?
- Does mapping your usual work activity into TRAMmCPD show that you are in fact developing your practice and it has developed into CPD?

If the answer to any of these questions is 'yes', it seems that your normal work practice has indeed made the transition into CPD. It can therefore be considered to be part of your CPD journey, which needs to be recorded.

Defining attribute 5 states that if you are really engaging in CPD, the learning continues beyond the initial CPD activity. We should therefore consider the importance of applying, recording, monitoring, measuring and sharing the impact of your learning (see Chapters 6–10).

How can you build support?
Professional development: finding support from other people

The importance of other people's influence on your professional development cannot be overestimated. For instance, some people may have modelled what you consider to be true professionalism and you may have strived to emulate the expertise of those individuals. You may have attributed aspects of your development to the direct influence of certain events and/or responses by service users/patients/students. You may also have experienced the personal and professional growth that has emerged from working in a collaborative and supportive learning team and through engaging in reflection, deliberation and debate of real-life issues.

The importance of others in professional development has been acknowledged by Webster-Wright (2009, p. 702). She suggests 'authentic professional learning' takes place over a long time and most usefully within a supportive learning community which may help you make sense of your learning, engaging you to work with others on real problems within your own professional practice (Boud & Middleton 2003, Burbank & Kauchak 2003, Oakes & Rogers 2007).

A study undertaken by Gunn and Goding (2009) explored the perceptions of community-based physiotherapists in relation to CPD they had undertaken. Interviews revealed that participants identified the benefits of discussing collaborative activities with peers, but acknowledged that the value of this type of CPD was often unappreciated, with many preferring to look to those they perceived as 'experts' for advice. This could be why, despite much of the evidence suggesting the importance of a range of learning activities for CPD, people often revert to considering attendance at courses and conferences as the only real way to learn and develop new skills. Based on this research, Gunn and Goding suggested there was a need for physiotherapists to further develop opportunities to collaborate in order to maximise potential CPD opportunities.

Collaboration is particularly important but can present a challenge, especially if you are a lone worker, a sole practitioner in a team, someone who feels isolated within a large team, or in a more rural location. In this type of situation, proactively locating or building your own professional support networks (for example, mentorship or learning communities) can be helpful to support your professional socialisation and engagement in CPD (HCPC 2015, RCOT 2017, Lawson 2018, Lawson & Tempest 2019).

You may find professional support in a variety of ways (both face to face and virtual) which are not confined to work environments (Alsop 2013, Playfoot & Hall 2018). Playfoot and Hall (2018, p. 14) state:

> Social learning gives the learner the power to initiate, manage and progress their own learning, on their own terms, whilst at the same time benefiting from other learners… Most of what we learn at work and elsewhere comes from engaging in networks where people co-create, collaborate and share knowledge, fully participating and actively engaging, driving and guiding their learning through whatever topics will help them improve.

Making the most of everyday opportunities to learn from others, discuss practice, reflect, observe each other and practise together may help your ongoing professional and ethical development, whilst increasing your confidence in your own practice (Lawson 2018).

Outside the workplace, there are increasing opportunities to learn from, and interact with, others. Access to social media, e-learning, virtual technologies, resources and platforms provided through professional organisations are making it easier to find support, which can enable you to network, learn, develop, reflect and share knowledge.

Suggestions for ways to build professional support networks which could also contribute to your CPD

- Make the most of opportunities to talk with others (online or face to face)
- Volunteer for a professional body/charity/specialist section or organisation
- Engage in journal clubs (online or face to face)
- Organise or join lunchtime learning events
- Attend local events for professionals and/or focusing on a condition you are interested in
- Identify mentorship opportunities (as a mentor/mentee)
- Join online chats/support groups (e.g. search for hashtags such as #OTalk #WeAHPs #PhysioTalk)

You may find further ideas in Chapter 2 and throughout this book.

The challenge with social learning in any format, is to recognise the potential for learning not only for intellectual interest and stimulation but also to be critical learners able to assess the quality of what is being learnt, document, reflect, evaluate the content and apply in practice for their CPD (Lawson & Hearle 2019a, 2019b).

Professional development: developing a learning culture

Although it is an essential aspiration, delivering high-quality health care in a complex organisation like the NHS or a Local Authority can be fraught with difficulty (Øvretveit 2009, 2011). Within such diverse and complex communities, conflicting goals (such as the need for continued quality improvement versus the need to balance increasing costs with shrinking budgets) are compounded by even greater complexities involving human factors. To manage service delivery within this complex system, it is essential that the NHS recruits and retains skilled, motivated staff who are able to respond to, and deliver on, the changes required. Continuing professional development (CPD) can enable this workforce to be created (HCPC 2019b, NMC 2019, Broughton & Harris 2019, NHS 2019).

Within many organisations there is a history of tick-box auditing, both imposed by the organisation and internally developed as part of departmental procedures. This tendency may be further driven by regulatory audits imposed by the HCPC or NMC and the implementation of systems such as the Knowledge and Skills Framework (KSF). Frank, Snell, et al. (2010) suggest that this focus on competencies and tick-boxes supports a reductionist approach to practice, which emphasises achieving minimum standards rather than pursuing best practice.

This is evident in the practice of departmental staff where path dependency features significantly and influences every part of practice. When this is a predominant characteristic, it is unsurprising that CPD is also presented as a tick-box activity, rather than something which is actively embraced by the team and organisation. This dependency upon previously adopted patterns of measurement can make it difficult for employees to think creatively and fully embrace the whole ethos of CPD. Instead they rely on a range of individual components (Rickles, Hawe & Shell 2007, Health Foundation 2010). This can still be seen today where CPD is often talked about in terms of 'doing CPD' and requiring the compliance of the individual, rather than the desire for engagement in CPD (Hearle & Lawson 2019) and the creation of conditions to facilitate engagement.

Webster-Wright (2009) highlights the need for learning to be contextualised in order to become 'authentic', encouraging individuals in organisations to actively engage in, rather than passively comply with, CPD. However, she also acknowledges the conflict in current research theory (which asserts the need for professional learning to take place in context, in real-life situations) with current practice where professional development is regulated, measured and relies heavily on formal training, rather than valuing authentic experiences.

As part of her doctoral research Lawson (2018) carried out a literature review which highlighted that working within a team in which learning appears to be embedded as a natural part of everyday practice, inherent in conversations, meetings and interactions where management and organisational support are explicit (Myers, Schaefer & Coudron 2017, Lloyd, Pfeiffer, et al. 2014), appears to facilitate recognition of, engagement in and the application of learning in practice. Fostering a learning culture within the workplace where informal and incidental learning are deliberately encouraged and recognised by the individual, their team, management and organisation (Marsick & Watkins 2015, p. 12.) may also lead to better outcomes for service users.

Organisational learning theory helps to provide an understanding of how such a learning environment can be developed. According to Garvin, Edmondson and Gino (2008 p. 1), a learning organisation is 'made up of employees skilled at creating, acquiring and transferring knowledge' for the benefit of themselves and the organisation. Garvin et al. argue that 'learning organisations' are able to adapt much more quickly to fast-changing environments and situations, and this is vital for the rapidly changing and evolving health and social care sectors.

Wang and Ahmed (2003) suggest that reciprocal learning can be achieved if the organisation appreciates and fosters the development of those individuals who work within it. This is supported by Garvin et al. (2008, p. 3), who identify this as one of the three building blocks of a learning organisation, alongside the need for 'concrete learning processes and practices, together with leadership behaviour that provides reinforcement'.

As a novice health and care professional, you may not have the authority to create such a learning organisation, but you do need to understand how you can work within one or influence decisions. If you are a leader in the organisation, however, it could be your responsibility to develop a learning culture and Garvin et al. (2008) suggest ways in which this can be achieved.

Firstly, it is important to foster a supportive setting for learning. This may mean ensuring that your team feel comfortable expressing their opinions or concerns and encouraging them to accept and value different ideas. This will enable your team to be more creative and push boundaries or take positive risks in their practice and create an environment where errors are discussed and resolved rather than hidden.

Garvin et al. (2008) also highlight the need to remove all the attention normally placed on accomplishing tasks and instead give permission for reflection. This could be facilitated by using small team activities either within specialist areas or with an initial focus on more generic issues of relevance to all, especially within teams where there are large numbers of members in disparate areas. It is acknowledged that removing the emphasis on accomplishment can be hard to achieve when the mandatory requirements mean that application in practice must be evidenced.

The second stage, according to Garvin et al. (2008), is to create effective learning processes and practices. Creative thinking maximises skills and knowledge across all areas and could produce excellent learning opportunities without negatively influencing the budget. Within your team, ask members to consider all the ways in which you could support new learning without missing long periods of core role time or ways in which you can create income opportunities for your area. Remember, allowing some time for positive learning experiences may increase staff retention and productivity and lead to more effective practice in the long term (Van den Broeck, Vansteenkiste, et al. 2008, Schaufeli & Bakker 2004).

Lack of appropriate and timely feedback can be a major flaw in an organisation's culture. Often, formal feedback regarding the outcome from CPD can be limited to documenting whether those objectives set in appraisal/professional development review have been met. Objectives set through this process may not be recorded appropriately, as true objectives (i.e. identifying specific outcomes), and may instead reflect passive requirements that can be ticked off (e.g. 'attend a course on mindfulness'). It is therefore important that employers advise employees about the importance of objectives and how to set, record, monitor and measure them. In particular, CPD objectives should reflect expected outcomes in practice (HCPC 2015, NMC 2019, Hearle & Lawson 2019). These outcomes can subsequently be fed back into the system much more effectively to develop quality of practice or, alternatively, cease those interventions which have little or no evidence base. Appropriate and timely feedback on CPD is essential for engagement (Hearle & Lawson 2019) and a core goal of clinical governance and prudent healthcare (Welsh Government 2019).

In addition, CPD within the department should be extended beyond the individual by ensuring dissemination of learning. This will allow the outcome (e.g. greater knowledge and skill) to be fed back into the wider system, enabling others and the organisation as a whole to benefit from the learning. This is part of the process of developing a learning organisation (Edmonson & Moingeon 1998, see below). It is also considered good practice from a financial perspective. One of the unintended consequences of the elevated status of CPD has been to place additional pressure on training budgets at a time when financial resources are limited. Greater input of CPD learning into the department/wider organisation maximises the potential effectiveness of individual CPD and may reduce expenditure on training/development and unnecessary duplication.

Finally, those of you who are aspiring leaders and wish to develop a learning culture should make sure that you question and challenge viewpoints in a constructive and supportive manner and openly welcome new ideas. Within a positive learning culture, staff also need to be supported to apply new knowledge, try out new skills and evaluate the outcome. Introducing a successful CPD strategy should, in theory, promote effectiveness and – through this – patient safety.

The National Advisory Group on the Safety of Patients in England (NAGSPE 2013) emphasised that the growth and development of staff providing care must be supported and should be a prime goal for health organisations if patient safety was to be achieved. They further stated that 'improvement requires a system of support' (NAGSPE 2013, p. 4) where capacity building was a 'core resourced objective'. The authors stressed the need to remove fear, describing it as 'toxic to both safety and improvement' (p. 4). They continued to highlight how poorly informed staff are more likely to become defensive in their practice and fear itself can cause anxiety, mistakes and a fear of reporting incidents. This is probably why the group's first recommendation was to 'continually and forever reduce patient harm by embracing wholeheartedly an ethic of learning' (NAGSPE 2013, p. 5). Learning from CPD includes the need to learn from our mistakes. It also means that staff (particularly those responsible for managing systems) need to master qualities such as leadership and learn skills (such as improvement science) that are required for successful change.

In order to support and advance learning from CPD, effective supervision is essential. This is addressed in greater depth in Chapter 9 but it is important at this point to emphasise the importance of providing a sound supervision strategy in relation to creating a learning culture.

Supervision gives individual staff 'Accountability' (facilitating safe and effective practice) and 'Support and Learning' (O'Neill 2004) and is now a required part of practice. Youngstrom (2009) and the Royal College of Occupational Therapists (COT 2010, 2015) state that the main aim of supervision is to achieve safe and effective service delivery which is of a high quality. For supervision to be beneficial, RCOT (COT 2010, 2015) and Strong (2009) also highlight the need for it to be conducted in a safe and supportive manner, as it has been found that fear and lack of trust result in more mistakes and less reporting (Dixon-Woods 2010).

In their study of allied health professionals, Strong, Kavanagh, et al. (2003) found that supervision can help to increase job satisfaction, effectiveness and clinical reasoning whilst at the same time preventing stress and burnout, two factors associated with poor patient safety (Olinky 2009). This was supported by Kavanagh, Spence, et al. (2003) who found positive benefits in terms of clinical effectiveness and staff morale. Strong, Kavanagh, et al. (2003) also identified organisational benefits of supervision, with staff developing a more grounded understanding of the organisational culture and practice and a stronger sense of identity. This understanding of the cultural and systems complexities of an organisation are considered essential in helping to ensure patient safety (NAGSPE 2013).

Developing your case for CPD

In order to develop an effective case for creating or engaging in CPD, it is important to be aware of the drivers and include them in any case you put forward. For example, your line manager is more likely to agree that you should set up a new learning group within your organisation if you can assure them of the benefits it will offer the local service and stakeholders. Your peers, on the other hand, may need to be reassured that the learning group will help their own professional development and can be used to provide evidence of their own progress.

The template below may help you to prepare and present your case accordingly. This is not a definitive case but it includes suggestions to get you started and it can be adapted according to what you wish to achieve. It is important to note that you do not need to complete every section of the template for every activity, as all applications will be different. There may also be bespoke templates for specific events available from the event organisers and it may be worth checking this out. Remember that whatever you are trying to do or attend must be seen to be value for money. The more it costs, the greater the perceived value you will need to demonstrate. You may find that there are training grants available from your organisation, professional body, government and charities.

Table 3.2 Business case for CPD activity

Business Case for Continuing Professional Development
Name: Area of practice: e.g. Podiatry
Details of the CPD Activity/Event
• What are you proposing to attend/set up? • What are the aims of the activity/event?
Benefits for yourself
• How will this activity/event help you to meet your PDR/Appraisal objectives? • How will it increase your knowledge and skills? • How will it contribute to your career and professional development? (Consider this across the four Pillars of Practice identified above.)
Benefits for service users/stakeholders
• How will you apply your learning? • What outcomes are you hoping it will influence for your service users (e.g. greater evidence for the intervention or discontinuation of intervention)?
Benefits for the team
• How will you ensure that this activity/event benefits other members of your team, e.g. how will you share what you learn with them? • Could it streamline processes for them or make their role easier?
Benefits for the organisation
• What are the goals of the organisation for which you work? • How could your proposal fit with these goals (e.g. potential to lead to shorter discharge times)?
Other additional benefits
• Does the activity/event link to wider strategic plans and/or policies? • Does it link with the goals for your profession? • Why? (Provide some context for this application, e.g. social prescribing is an important consideration in primary care.)
Details of any resource/time costs to the organisation
• What physical resources will you need (e.g. a meeting room for 20 people once a month, photocopying?) • How long will you be away from work? • How much are you asking for (full cost/contribution/time onl/travel expenses)?

Details of your own contribution to the cost of resources/time
● How much time will you be contributing and how? ● Have you applied for any grants to support this attendance? If so how much are the grants expected to contribute?
How, where and when will the learning be shared with others?
● How will you disseminate your learning to your colleagues? ● Will you present the application of this new learning to your organisation? ● Do you plan to publish in a professional journal/newsletter? ● Might this have international implications for dissemination?

Case study: Sally reflects upon the meaning of CPD

In the first two chapters we introduced Sally, an occupational therapist who attended a two-day conference part-funded by her employer, where she went to several sessions with no forethought or planning. One of the activities she has been participating in is a journal club where they have been discussing the meaning of CPD engagement. Following this, Sally has begun to realise that she may need to take a different approach to meet the HCPC standards for CPD.

Sally is enjoying working in mental health as part of her rotation but is concerned that she is being asked to consider the use of Cognitive Behavioural Therapy (CBT) as an intervention, despite having no real experience with CBT. Sally has a quick look on the internet to locate some credible websites, with video footage illustrating the application of CBT, as she knows this will help her to remember things more easily (self-directed learning). She also retrieves her handouts and lecture notes from university about how this intervention can be used by occupational therapists. Using a mind map (see Chapter 7), she has formulated a summary of the core aspects, including an overview of the main principles of CBT. She realises that, although she can apply the principles, she needs further training in order to become proficient in its use.

During her investigations she discovers that there is a 12-month training programme coming up in London next year. She also sees a two-day programme run by the local mental health special interest group, which is scheduled in three weeks' time (a formal training opportunity). This will be at the right level and she can fund it herself if her manager will allow her to take the time off work. The course in London is very specialised and expensive. Although she would love to do something like this, she decides that it is more appropriate if she specialises in mental health at a later date.

In supervision her manager asks her to put together a case to attend the two-day training in which she is expected to outline the benefits to herself, service users, the team and wider organisation. Her manager also suggests that Sally finds out more about her strengths and preferred learning style to ensure that she makes the most from any learning activities.

Tasks

The following tasks may enable you to view CPD in a more creative and expansive way and identify how you can make the most of all potential learning opportunities to engage in your CPD:

1. Reflect on your current attitude to CPD and highlight areas that may need addressing.

2. Reflect on how you recognise when you are learning something new which may have the potential to become CPD (see 'How do you know when your normal work practice becomes CPD?' above).

3. Consider ways in which you could be more proactive with your learning. Think about how they could be integrated within your everyday practice

4. What day-to-day opportunities are there within your workplace? Develop one learning opportunity for your team, and encourage other team members to consider how this could contribute to their own CPD.

5. Map your own progress to a career/learning development framework (see Table 3.1).

6. Make a list of elements that you could contribute towards the culture of learning within your team/organisation

7. Read on to Chapter 4 to understand more about yourself and ways to develop further.

4

Recognising your strengths and developing your preferred learning style

There is no such thing as 'one size fits all' in continuing professional development. This is acknowledged by gatekeepers of CPD such as the HCPC (2017a), which emphasises the value of accessing a variety of activities to strengthen your portfolio. Chapter 2 explored the range and value of some of these activities to help you find the most appropriate form of CPD to suit your requirements. However, there are other critical factors when planning and selecting activities for your CPD journey.

Chapter 3 explored the concept of CPD engagement which highlighted some of the reasons why identifying your strengths and preferred learning styles may be important. The first part of this chapter provides examples of tools to help you identify your own preferred learning style, and suggests ways to maximise your learning according to each style and context. The second part will focus on how to apply these learning skills and explore ways of applying them in practice.

Tasks at the end of the chapter will enable you to explore your strengths and most effective learning styles, and you will be given references and links for tools to help you do this.

What do we mean by individual strengths and preferred learning styles and how might awareness of these factors help your CPD?

In order to fully engage in CPD, the ability to self-direct your own learning is crucial. In Chapter 3 we explored the importance of taking responsibility for your own CPD. McClelland (1985) discussed the importance of measuring motivation and achievement in order to identify the level of self-directedness of an individual using the Need for Achievement (nAch) Test. To put nAch in context, it is useful to consider the work of Penman (2014), an occupational therapist, who explored factors influencing approaches to CPD in the research for her doctorate. Penman (2014) discovered that, in order to engage, individuals must show 'readiness' to be self-directed learners. This involves taking responsibility for your own learning and being aware of your own learning needs.

If we compare ourselves with colleagues, friends or family, it becomes clear that we all have very specific approaches towards activities (whether work or leisure) and the types of roles we perform. For example, some people will be motivated by sporting and team activities or competitions; others will enjoy more individual, quiet activities such as reading or baking. The same applies to learning.

Most people are born with the capacity to learn new things. During our lives, and throughout our education, most of us find some things more interesting or easier to learn than others. For instance, some people easily pick up the words to songs, whereas others do not 'hear' the words but easily recognise the tune. Some can read a set of instructions and instinctively know how to assemble a piece of furniture, while others have to look at the diagrams or may even be able to assemble the item just by looking at the parts and the final picture. An individual's preferred choice of learning style does not make that one person any 'brighter' than another, and there is no style that suits all. The trick is to recognise the learning style that works best for you, in a variety of situations, and develop strategies to improve your learning using other modalities.

When identifying your strengths and preferred learning style, another consideration is the learning context. This can also be a personal preference. For example, some people learn best through hands-on practice and may therefore find role-play situations or work-based learning most appropriate. Others may learn and be able to apply information just from attending a seminar or lecture and find role-play stressful and unhelpful. Context is also important when considering the learning required. If someone needs to acquire new information about a condition, for example, attending a lecture, conference or reading a book or article may be enough. However, if the CPD is aimed at learning a new skill or applying a new intervention, the learning may have to take place in a simulated or work-based setting, regardless of preferred learning style.

Before you read the next section about how to find out about your strengths and preferred learning style, it is important to be aware of some of the pitfalls or limitations. Although learning styles analysis tools are readily available and frequently utilised, there is much debate about their actual usefulness and there are sometimes risks associated with isolating a particular learning style. Learning style tests/recommendations should not be seen as a simple solution to a complex issue such as learning (Learning and Skills Research Centre 2004). We have already acknowledged that there are several factors, such as context and type of learning, which may influence a preferred style of learning. We have also identified the need to ensure that you do not rely solely on the results of your preferred style, highlighting the need to identify strategies to improve those areas less favourable to you.

Krätzig and Arbuthnott (2006) also demonstrated that learning strengths and preferences are not always the same. For example, it may be suggested in a test that your strength is 'read/write learning' but in fact you enjoy attending lectures because it helps to clarify your understanding, whereas reading a book may not. This may explain students' confusion when looking at their results from specific tests and the apparent conflict between their strengths and preferences.

The next section examines some of the most commonly available tools that can help you recognise your learning style strengths and preferences and how you can make the best use of this information. We have included these in the new edition of this book because many people have suggested that they form a useful starting point for engaging in CPD. We would therefore advise readers to exercise caution, using such tools as a guide but not relying so heavily on their results that it distorts their enjoyment and pursuit of CPD. If you choose to try out one of the more structured/standardised tests identified below, you should look at what some researchers say about these tests when assessing their credibility. You can then use this information to help you to critically reflect upon how you might use this information when considering your results. This will promote a more evidence-based approach to your reflection, as advocated by Newton and Miah (2017).

How can you identify your learning style strength or preference?

One simple (and free) way to ascertain your preferred learning style is to undertake a written (and preferably critical) reflection. Following a specific model (see Chapter 7), you should reflect upon a recent activity where you felt you learnt something. Consider which elements you enjoyed and found helpful in terms of learning, and which you found less effective. Also, try to analyse why some elements helped you to learn, and why others did not. Once you have done this, consider in what contexts these factors might change.

Mind mapping (see Chapter 7) may help you organise your thoughts to produce a more visual representation of your thoughts and reflections.

If you prefer a more structured method to identify your learning strengths, there are various standardised tools available. Some of the most common include:

- VARK (Visual–Auditory–Read/Write–Kinaesthetic) test
- Honey and Mumford Learning Styles Questionnaire
- Kolb's Learning Styles Inventory
- nAch (Need for Achievement)

The VARK test

The VARK test (Fleming & Mills 1992) consists of a series of 16 questions that explore learning style preferences in given situations. Each question has four possible answers and you are required to select the answer that describes how you would be most likely to behave. Here is an example of the type of question you might find in the VARK test (VARK 2019):

You have finished a competition or test and would like some feedback…
a. Using a written description of your results
b. Using a graph showing what you have achieved

c. From somebody who talks it through with you

d. Using examples from what you have done.

At the end of the test, you simply count up the numbers of As, Bs, Cs and Ds to find your preferred style of learning, as follows:

- Visual learners (learn best from visual cues and pictures)
- Auditory learners (learn best from auditory cues, lectures and talking things through)
- Read/write learners (learn best from making lists and notes, and being given handouts)
- Kinaesthetic/tactile learners (learn best from doing things and carrying out activities).

Once you have matched your score to your learning preference, there are explanations of those things that each type of learner finds useful. Some people may be very biased towards one particular style, while others may be quite close in two or more categories. The VARK team stress that, although your score may indicate one preference, this only refers to your learning, which may be influenced by strategies you have developed during your life. It does not suggest how you undertake other things (such as work) or how you behave in relation to other people. The test is free and you can access other learning support media through the website www.vark-learn.com.

The Kolb Learning Style Inventory and Honey and Mumford learning styles

Kolb (1984) suggests that there are four main stages in learning:

1. Concrete experience, in which the individual encounters a new experience or situation or reinterprets an existing experience
2. Reflective observation, in which the individual reflects on the experience, noting differences between the experience and their understanding
3. Abstract conceptualisation, in which the reflection stimulates a new idea or modification
4. Active experimentation, in which learning is applied and evaluated.

In Kolb's cycle, no one stage is more important than any other so the learner can enter the cycle at any point. However, he argues that the most effective learning occurs when the individual moves through all four stages.

As in the VARK test, Kolb believes that individuals tend to prefer one learning style above another. This preference is influenced by various factors, including the person's social environment, their educational experiences and their own cognitive make-up. However, he also emphasises that this does not provide an excuse to make sole use of that preferred style. Instead individuals must work on those areas where learning is less comfortable in order to gain a more rounded and effective learning experience. To help you explore different types of learning, Kolb offers a specific Learning Style Inventory, which is available at: https://learningfromexperience.com/themes/kolb-learning-style-inventory-lsi/

There is also the Honey and Mumford (1992) Learning Styles Questionnaire which reflects the principles of Kolb's learning cycle. Honey and Mumford give you the choice of completing one of two questionnaires – one of 40 or one of 80 statements. Whichever one you choose, you are asked to answer as honestly as possible by agreeing or disagreeing with each statement. Once you have completed the questionnaire, you can transfer your responses to a grid, which will give you a score out of 20 for each of the following learning style categories:

1. The Activist: you learn by doing, or by having an experience
2. The Reflector: you learn by reviewing the experience from a number of perspectives
3. The Theorist: you need to understand the underpinning theories, drawing conclusions from the experience
4. The Pragmatist: you learn by seeing how to put into practice and planning the next steps.

Once you have highlighted your preferred style/s, and those which are more problematic for you, Honey and Mumford provide descriptors and action plans for each one.

Maintaining a self-directed approach

Having identified your strengths, preferred learning style and selected an area you wish to know more about in order to improve your knowledge and skills, how do you bring all this together in order to apply your learning in practice?

Whilst it is useful to be aware of your strengths and learning preferences and apply them, these are not the only factors involved in engaging in CPD. A number of external factors are considered in Chapter 3, but one core element of being a professional is the internal factor of maintaining a desire to know more (Bargagliotti 2012). This is supported by Penman (2014) with her research into the link between readiness for self-directed learning and CPD engagement. Penman (2014, p. 1) states that this readiness is influenced by:

> 'beliefs or attitudes to learning, the degree of metacognitive awareness [of themselves] as learners, and personal definitions of competence to practice, with experience in supervision of allied health students and occupational therapists, and years employed'.

This idea of self-directedness relates to all aspects of the CPD process, which is discussed broadly in Chapter 3 and explored in greater depth in Chapters 6–10. The first step is to identify your own learning development plan; and the best way to do this is to consider and document your aspirational career pathway or immediate goals for professional development. Using your profession's career development framework can be invaluable in identifying your current skills and knowledge and those you wish to develop further. One example is that developed by the Royal College of Occupational Therapists (2017) based on the four Pillars of Practice: Professional Practice; Facilitation of Learning; Leadership; Evidence, Research and Development. For other examples of career and development frameworks see Chapter 3, Table 3.1. Your professional development and learning goals may be most effectively articulated by generating Specific, Measurable, Achievable, Realistic and Timely (SMART) objectives (see example below).

Your SMART objectives should be negotiated and agreed with your supervisor or as part of your regular appraisal. You may also wish to discuss your plans with your mentor prior to this (see Chapters 6, 9 and 10). You can either do this by writing a set of objectives or use a more structured tool, such as a learning contract (see Chapter 7). Remember, whatever you decide, you must write the objectives as something you want to achieve rather than something you are going to do.

For example, 'To spend time with the community rehabilitation team by the end of the month' is a passive activity that may not result in any learning.

It would be better to reword it as: 'Through a written reflection, I will demonstrate a comprehensive understanding of the role and scope of the community rehabilitation team and compare it with my role in social care. This is to be achieved within the next four weeks and validated by my line manager.'

This objective requires your active engagement, leading to a measurable outcome. To make it more detailed, you could indicate the evidence you will provide to show you have gained comprehensive understanding.

For health and social care professionals, the main purpose of CPD is to foster improvement in care for service users (HCPC 2017a, Broughton & Harris 2019). The fourth HCPC standard requires you to provide evidence to demonstrate how you have achieved this through CPD (HCPC 2017a). The various ways you might apply your learning in practice are explored in depth in Chapter 8.

Case study:
Sally investigates her preferred learning styles and strengths

Sally decides to explore her preferred learning style and strengths, as suggested by her colleague who attended the TRAMmCPD workshop (Chapter 2). Sally decides to carry out some self-directed informal internet research, where she finds a range of resources that may help her identify her strengths and preferred learning style. She is particularly drawn to the resources available on the VARK website (Fleming & Mills 1992) and she would also like to try Honey and Mumford (1992) because she knows their questionnaire is based on Kolb's (1984) Learning Cycle, a learning framework with which she is already familiar.

Having completed the VARK test, Sally realises her strengths are primarily as a kinaesthetic learner, with visual tendencies. She then completes the Honey and Mumford Learning Styles Questionnaire, which reveals that she predominantly favours an Activist approach and indicates that her Reflector category is very low and this is an area she needs to work on.

Now that she is aware of her strengths and preferred learning style, Sally understands that she learns best by 'doing' and this will need to be her focus, where possible, when planning the best ways to learn new skills. Her investigations suggest that she will learn best by attending interactive workshops, shadowing and work-based learning, rather than attending lectures or presentations.

Whichever CPD activity she chooses, she now knows that she must find ways to participate actively, as sitting listening in lectures and presentations does not stimulate her ability to learn. As an Activist (based on the Honey and Mumford questionnaire), she realises she needs assistance to increase such opportunities for practical learning and participation.

This does not mean that Sally should only consider practical activities for her CPD, as this may not always be possible or practicable. For example, if Sally attends a lecture, she may need to consider strategies, such as making notes involving practical application to real-life people she is working with, or has worked with, rather than simply recording the main points from the lecture.

The results from the Honey and Mumford questionnaire remind Sally that reflective skills are not her strength, and she needs to find ways to encourage and challenge her skills of reflection. Previously, she has used Gibbs' reflective cycle (1988), which she remembers was easy to use and understand. All her identified strengths and preferred learning style information can be used when considering her future learning needs, and this will provide a good focus for her CPD over the next few months. Happy with the progress she has made, she decides to discuss her plans at her next supervision.

Tasks

The following tasks will enable you to explore your strengths, revise and consolidate your most effective learning styles and help you use this information to engage more effectively with CPD:

1. Have a look at the suggested learning styles websites to see if any of the tests or questionnaires are useful to you. If not, investigate further examples.

2. Complete one of the preferred learning style tests or questionnaires to see what they suggest about you. Do you agree?

3. What are your learning needs, in addition to your strengths and preferred learning styles identified above?

4. Arrange a meeting with your supervisor or mentor to explore what actions you can take as a result of the above findings.

5. Consider what you could do to foster a conducive CPD environment within your work environment. Discuss your ideas with your manager if this is something you are not able to implement yourself.

6. If you are a manager reading this chapter, consider how you might alter your management or teaching style to reflect individual learning needs within each of the categories of Kolb and Honey and Mumford.

7. Read Chapter 5 to find out more about the TRAMm Model and its tools and how they can help you.

5

Introduction to the TRAMm model

This chapter introduces mechanisms for strategic CPD using TRAMmCPD. It explains why the TRAMm model and its associated tools were developed and how they can help you plan and execute your professional development. The chapter has been updated to include recent changes to the TRAMm Model based on the outcomes of our research. It outlines the main components (stations) of the model and explores how the model and its tools can be used, illustrated with a case study and working examples.

Tasks at the end of the chapter encourage you to identify core learning needs in relation to your personal and professional development using TRAMmCPD. You can also consider how you might use TRAMmCPD to provide a framework for your professional development.

Why do we need a model for CPD?

The CPD Audit Report (HCPC 2019b) suggests that those who undertake CPD are less likely to find themselves the subject of a complaint or concern and are more likely to be, or become, reflective practitioners. The TRAMm Model was designed after initial investigations of potential structures for professional development support groups revealed a scarcity of frameworks to guide the process of CPD at an individual level.

The importance of CPD engagement

In Chapter 3 we saw that it is part of our professional responsibility to undertake CPD; but undertaking CPD is not enough in itself. Certain factors also need to be in place to enable us to engage with CPD. What do we mean by the concept of engagement in relation to CPD?

Much has been written on the subject of worker/employee engagement in CPD; yet the meaning of CPD engagement remains less than clear, as we saw in Chapter 3. As a reminder, the criteria for CPD engagement, according to Hearle and Lawson (2019), are:

1. When an individual is engaged, the CPD activity is self-initiated and undertaken voluntarily, rather than purely because it is a mandatory requirement.

2. The motivation to undertake the activity can be intrinsic or extrinsic. The individual feels rewarded either intrinsically (e.g. through their own enjoyment) or extrinsically (e.g. through promotion), while undertaking or after undertaking the CPD activity.

3. The knowledge and skills gained via the CPD are embraced and applied in practice for the benefit of the organisation and service user/s.

4. Learning is recorded, evaluated and shared with others.

5. Learning is shown to continue beyond the initial CPD activity.

Although the TRAMm Model was initially designed as a CPD guide for individuals, to give them the best opportunity to engage with their own professional development, the organisation in which they work must also accept some responsibility for supporting its employees. This is reflected in the most recent *Principles for Continuing Professional Development and Lifelong Learning in Health and Social Care* (Broughton & Harris 2019) where the responsibilities of stakeholders are outlined.

Simpson (2009) identified the availability of resources as an especially important factor in encouraging employee engagement, especially as CPD is usually undertaken in the workplace. However, despite the continuing emphasis on the importance of CPD in practice, anecdotal evidence from managers and practitioners suggests that the resources (including money and time) available for CPD in organisations appear to have been reduced in recent years. Not surprisingly, this has subsequently appeared to result in a lack of engagement in CPD (AMRC 2010, Gould et al. 2007).

The rise in employee workload, and the individual guilt associated with taking time away from critical patient care, are other factors thought to result in disengagement from CPD (O'Sullivan 2003, 2006). In contrast, those employers considered to be 'learning organisations' (O'Sullivan 2006) encourage employees to engage with their own CPD by supporting them and offering them opportunities to identify and address their learning and development needs. In learning organisations, evidence-based practice is encouraged and processes such as appraisal, supervision, mentorship and preceptorship (see Chapters 9 and 10) help to create and maintain a supportive environment. If individuals are encouraged in this way, they are likely to be more engaged by their work, which in turn stimulates a drive to learn more in order to keep improving the quality of their work. CPD engagement thus becomes a virtuous cycle. Having said this, it is important to acknowledge that the opposite may sometimes occur – for instance, when burnout in an existing role leads to an extrinsic desire for CPD, resulting in a change in career direction.

We are not saying that a lack of time and money means that you cannot be expected to engage in CPD; but we are acknowledging a mutual responsibility, as CPD clearly offers shared benefits for both the individual and organisation. Several chapters in this book explore how you and your organisation can work together in this way. Effective CPD, where individuals are fully engaged with their own professional development, has been found to correlate with a higher quality of care for the service user (DH 2001, AHPP 2003, AMRC 2010, HCPC 2015). Service users are bound to benefit when CPD is undertaken by individual staff members motivated by a need to know more and to find evidence supporting the effectiveness (or otherwise) of different types of patient intervention.

It is also widely accepted that work engagement leads to greater job satisfaction and therefore less chance of burnout (Maslach et al, 2001, Van der Broeck et al. 2008, NHS Staff Council 2009, Schaufeli & Bakker 2004). If a person is engaged in their work, they have a drive to know more and to strive for best practice, which is furthered by their engagement in CPD. Hence, it is also likely that CPD engagement will result in greater learner satisfaction and job satisfaction and subsequently in higher retention of staff (O'Sullivan 2006, AMRC 2010).

A further consequence of full engagement in CPD is the wider dissemination of learning (AMRC 2010) and hence the potential for the learning to benefit more service users. The potential benefits apply to service users treated by the individual and their immediate colleagues and also to those treated by a much wider range of professionals within organisations, by means of publication in peer-reviewed journals and presentations at national or international conferences.

Different approaches to CPD

It is not possible to design a CPD programme to fit every single person, as we all have different approaches to our learning and skills development. However, a model or framework can help to draw the necessary components of CPD together into a cohesive whole, providing a structure for this complex and often misunderstood process, while respecting the unique requirements of each individual.

Before exploring how the TRAMm Model can assist you in planning and organising your CPD in a more strategic and efficient way, it may be helpful to examine the approach you usually take to the process of CPD. Consider the following examples, which portray a range of approaches to CPD. As you read them, think about which one most closely matches your own style. You may find that more than one applies to you, but be honest about which one fits you best.

Example 5.1 The ostrich

George is a radiographer, who has been qualified for 22 years. He works in an English town at the local hospital. He is conscious that he has not 'done' any recent CPD and that radiographers are due to be audited by the HCPC later this year, but he is fairly certain he won't be one of the 'unlucky' ones. He therefore plans to keep his head down and worry about it if and when it happens.

Example 5.2 The procrastinator

Sarina is a Band 7 podiatrist, who works as part of the same older adult team as George. She knows that each time the podiatry audit comes around it could well apply to her. She has dutifully undertaken her CPD during each of the six years she has been qualified, usually attending courses following recommendations from her manager. She is aware that she hasn't started to make records in her portfolio, but often thinks about how to do it and plans to make a start 'next week'. Sadly, next week never seems to arrive.

Example 5.3 The bull in a china shop

Ben, a physiotherapist, has been qualified for nearly two years. He is very enthusiastic about his work and is always very busy in his role in the outpatients department of an inner-city hospital. He is keen to ensure that he stays as up-to-date as possible and is very conscientious about CPD. He is proud of the fact that he has already been on 13 short courses and conferences on a wide variety of topics (some in his own time) and has just lined up two more one-day refresher sessions over the next three months. He has two A4 lever-arch folders full of reflections, course notes and certificates. Although these files are not yet organised, he has a lot to show people if they ask to see his CPD records.

Example 5.4 The strategist

Janet has recently obtained a Band 5 Speech and Language Therapist post and is currently awaiting her final results before she can apply for her HCPC registration. Previously a healthcare assistant with no formal qualifications, Janet was keen to continue to work in a healthcare setting but in a more defined and professional role. After deciding that speech and language therapy was her chosen career path, she successfully completed the appropriate A-levels at evening classes, which enabled her to qualify for university. While awaiting the results of her final exams, she is continuing to plan her professional development. Having attended a TRAMmCPD workshop, she has consolidated her strategic skills at university, based on the HCPC standards, using TRAMmCPD. She is hoping to work with children and is currently focusing her CPD in this area, through volunteering at a local specialist school. This will mean that she is well placed to apply for relevant posts as they arise.

Which example resembles you most closely? Clearly, most of us would aspire to emulate Janet ('the strategist'). She is focused on her career path and takes a strategic approach to reaching her objectives. However, if you find yourself more closely resembling one of the others, you are by no means on your own – and this can be easily rectified.

For instance, if you are most like George ('the ostrich'), you need to take your head out of the sand and start to embrace CPD. Begin collating your portfolio, using the items you have already gathered. You should also think about those activities you have undertaken in the last 12 months that could be classed as CPD (see Chapter 2). Carry out a couple of reflections to evidence your learning and make an appointment with your line manager or supervisor to discuss some objectives to take you through to the next appraisal.

If you find you resemble Sarina ('the procrastinator'), find a file or an electronic portfolio structure. Then undertake a couple of reflections or look at evidencing the outcomes of this CPD via a case study. Think carefully about where you see your future direction and talk to your supervisor about the strategic direction of the organisation so that you can help initiate your own plans for any future CPD, rather than waiting to be told by your manager.

If you are like Ben ('the bull'), your enthusiasm is to be commended but you really need to start refining what you do and focus on quality rather than quantity. Set aside some time to go through all your reflections and certificates and get them organised into a portfolio. You could perhaps undertake one reflection on your CPD as a whole, to date. Then see if there are any themes arising from the CPD you have already done, and which CPD activities you think have been most useful. This should give you an idea of your future direction, and which aspects of CPD you should pursue.

Once you have a clear awareness of your current approach and have got to grips with what you have achieved to date, you need to consider how TRAMmCPD can provide a framework to help you understand ways to address your future development and learning needs.

What is TRAMmCPD?

TRAMmCPD consists of the TRAMm Model and its tools, the TRAMm Tracker and TRAMm Trail. The TRAMm Model has been developed as a dynamic, interactive model to facilitate a strategic approach to CPD (Hearle, Lawson & Morris 2016). CPD is now mandatory for health and care professionals, and this model uses an outcomes-based approach, in which aims are based on the CPD's likely impact, rather than simply 'doing' CPD for its own sake.

Although there have been many different approaches to CPD, research has revealed that none of them bring together all the HCPC's requirements into a coherent whole. The TRAMm Model was therefore initially designed to assist professionals registered with the HCPC to engage in and evidence CPD as part of their biennial registration process. However, the principles of this model are equally applicable for any individual who needs to continue their professional development, such as nurses (O'Keeffe 2016), doctors, lawyers and many other professionals.

The TRAMm Model is based on the fact that professionals not only need to learn new information and skills but must also plan their professional development, apply their newly acquired knowledge and skills within practice, measure their success (or otherwise), and share evidence of their practice with others. New knowledge not only adds value; it also provides the ability to deliver high-quality care. When knowledge is transferred into practice, it deepens the individual's ability to create, share, disseminate and present.

Continuing professional development is an individual journey that reflects the core unique qualities and skills of each practitioner. To be successful, it should be a strategic journey that is planned according to the individual's needs in relation to their professional practice and the organisation in which they work. It should contain a mixture of activities that reflect the strengths and preferred learning styles of the individual (see Chapters 2 and 4) and the type of knowledge or skill required in their practice. For example, there would be little point in simply reading a textbook if the main aim of the CPD was to develop your neurological handling skills. The textbook might help you acquire knowledge but could not replace actual practice in order to develop the skill itself. Undertaking activities alone does not constitute CPD. Instead, it is important that the individual applies what they have learnt from the activity/ies in practice, monitors their progress and success, before measuring the final outcome and readjusting their practice accordingly.

A Strategic Guide to Continuing Professional Development for Health and Care Professionals:
THE TRAMm Model

The TRAMm Model has been designed alongside tools (the TRAMm Tracker and TRAMm Trail) to provide a framework and encourage your engagement in CPD. Together, the Model and tools are known as TRAMmCPD. TRAMmCPD can be used by individuals and by the organisations in which they work. While individuals are more likely to use this to plan and record their CPD, organisations may choose to adopt TRAMmCPD as a corporate tool by which CPD is facilitated and measured. This is illustrated by the following example.

Example 5.5 The potential use of TRAMmCPD
Allyson is a physiotherapist who has recently read about TRAMmCPD in her colleague's professional body newsletter. She has accessed the website and downloaded the free TRAMmCPD tools and information about how to apply them. She has started an electronic portfolio, following the TRAMmCPD stations, and has begun to use the tools to record the details of her CPD. After taking this to a supervision session with her therapy lead, she has been asked to present TRAMmCPD to the team – so that all therapy professionals across the health board can adopt this as a framework to structure, present and measure their CPD.

What are the TRAMm Model stations?

In order to reflect the full CPD journey, the TRAMm Model is divided into five stations: 'Tell', 'Record', 'Apply', 'Monitor' and 'measure'. You will note that 'measure' is denoted by a lower-case 'm'. This is solely to differentiate it from 'Monitor' and in no way reflects the relative importance afforded to each station.

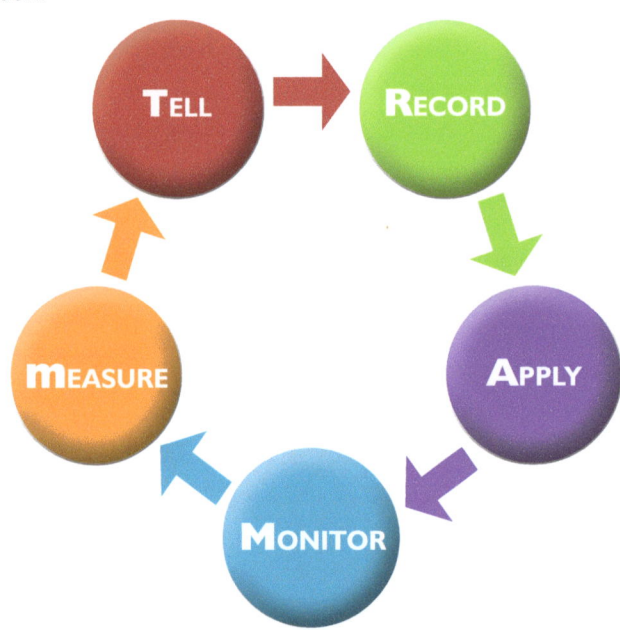

Figure 5.1 The TRAMm stations

Each of the five TRAMm stations is briefly summarised below. (They are explained in detail in Chapters 4–8.)

Station T (Tell, see Chapter 6): 'Tell' is about articulating and planning what you need or would like to learn (professional development planning), disseminating information about what you have learnt and developing your own learning community.

Station R (Record, see Chapter 7): 'Record' refers to the systematic documentation and evidence of what you have learnt, how you have applied your learning in practice and your reflections on the process, including what you need to learn next. It may also include the recording of outcomes and practice critique.

Station A (Apply, see Chapter 8): 'Apply' is how you have used and implemented your new learning, knowledge and/or skills in practice to benefit yourself, your service users and other stakeholders.

Station M (Monitor, see Chapter 9): 'Monitor' refers to keeping track of your development or reviewing your progress so you can alter your approach or change direction if you find that what you are doing is not meeting your learning needs.

Station m (measure, see Chapter 10): 'measure' means considering the impact of your learning and development on yourself and others, through tangible outcomes, such as achievement of goals, audit targets and success factors. Measurement does not need to be complex but does require validation in order to provide evidence of achievement.

Table 5.1 provides examples of possible activities within each of the stations. These lists are by no means exhaustive and you may well be able to add to them.

Table 5.1 Suggestions for entries included in the stations of the TRAMm Model stations

T – TELL (Chapter 6)	R – RECORD (Chapter 7)
● Informal/formal discussion with colleagues/Meetings	● Reflective logs
● Annual appraisals	● Mind Maps
● Planning in supervision	● Learning contracts
● Conferences/Courses/Presentations	● Publications
● Workshops/Team-building exercises	● Annual appraisal/supervision paperwork
● Training/Roadshows/Away days	● Case notes
● Sharing case studies/	● Social media
● Publications	● Professional development Portfolio
● Providing feedback from CPD	● Curriculum Vitae (CV)
● Social media/Email/Intranet/Internet	● TRAMm Tracker/Trail

A – APPLY (Chapter 8)	
• New knowledge is used in practice • Utilise a new skill • Implement a new intervention/way of working • Change in approach, values and/or behaviour • Use up-to-date evidence to inform practice	• Assess financial impact of your learning • Stop doing something/do something differently as a result of new knowledge • Introduce new policies, procedures, strategies, ways of working
M – MONITOR (Chapter 9)	**m – measure (Chapter 10)**
• Supervision • Mentorship • Annual appraisal/supervision process • Preceptorship or equivalent • Peer reviews • Self-monitoring through reflection	• Appraisal/Specific individualised goals achieved • Reflection/Skill acquisition and improvement • Using outcome measures/Performance indicators/ Audit/Regulation/Standards of proficiency • Peer review • Preceptorship • Undertaking research/quality improvement projects • Measuring cost effectiveness • Miscellaneous, e.g. Letters of Commendation, awards • Anecdotal, e.g. confidence, time

How does the TRAMm model work?

The TRAMm Model allows you to identify the gaps in your CPD, by reviewing each station and identifying those you still need to visit in order to maximise your engagement in CPD and its impact for yourself and all the stakeholders involved. Identifying gaps in your experience and knowledge enables you to seek and plan activities for your CPD. The TRAMm Model's flexible approach allows you to visit each station as and when appropriate. This is why it is depicted as a circle, rather than a linear series of stages. Although CPD usually starts with an activity, this is not always the case. For example, a discussion with a colleague or manager may trigger an idea that requires further exploration or training so that it can be effectively applied in practice.

The TRAMm Tracker and TRAMm Trail have been designed to assist you in recording and monitoring your CPD: the TRAMm Tracker allows you to record your CPD journey; and the

TRAMm Trail enables you to plan and analyse specific aspects of your CPD in greater detail (see Chapter 7 for full details of these tools). TRAMmCPD has been refined since its inception, following feedback from users and as a result of further research (Lawson 2018; Hearle and Lawson 2019, Lawson and Hearle 2019a, 2019b).

Why do you need TRAMmCPD?

The core reasons why TRAMmCPD can be a useful resource are:

1. It can encourage recognition of, engagement in and application of learning.
Visiting the TRAMm Model stations can help you to fully engage in CPD by becoming more aware when you are learning something which has the potential to become CPD and when you are using your learning in practice to benefit yourself and others.

2. It can help individuals maximise their professional potential.
TRAMmCPD can help you become (more) strategic and maximise your career potential. CPD can be a complex lifelong journey, which requires you to plan your career progression strategically, while at the same time meeting the needs of the organisation within which you work. TRAMmCPD encourages you to plot your journey, record your progress, apply your learning in practice and monitor and measure outcomes, while ensuring that you achieve a balance between your own needs and those of the service users you work with.

3. It can enable individuals to meet the HCPC standards for CPD.
TRAMmCPD can also help you meet the HCPC standards for CPD (HCPC 2017a). In the United Kingdom, most health and care professionals must be registered with their statutory body. For health and care professionals, the HCPC is commissioned by the government to regulate fitness to practise and provide standards of proficiency for each regulated profession. The aim is to ensure that all registrants practise lawfully, safely, skilfully and effectively. The HCPC also has a remit to ensure that all registrants undertake CPD, which must adhere to five specific standards (see Chapter 1). These CPD standards form part of a biennial audit process whereby registrants are required to demonstrate their ability to meet the standards and maintain ethical practice. Using the TRAMm Model, TRAMm Tracker and TRAMm Trail (TRAMmCPD) gives you a framework to facilitate your engagement in CPD and provide evidence of this process.

4. It can contribute to the creation of a learning organisation.
Although initially designed for individuals, TRAMmCPD can also be a useful resource for organisations and their managers because it offers a way of structuring CPD within the workplace and contributing to creation of a learning organisation. Within the pilot evaluation, some departments adopted TRAMmCPD to provide a consistent approach to CPD across the team, using the tools to monitor progress and facilitate discussion in supervision or appraisal sessions.

How can you use the TRAMm model?

Although the TRAMm Model is represented as a circular model, it is designed to be used as a dynamic framework, in which all stations are linked and can interact to provide a strategic approach to CPD.

The stations can be visited in any order, and can be visited more than once, or not at all, in relation to a single part of your CPD. Although not every part of your CPD will require you to visit every TRAMm station, within your total professional journey you should aim to include each of the five elements of TRAMm at regular intervals. The TRAMm Tracker can be used to help you identify those stations not yet visited or those you are avoiding, and this will help you monitor your CPD progress.

Example 5.6 Using the TRAMm Tracker

Mark is a radiographer. Six months ago, he went to a conference where he attended a seminar discussing a new way of undertaking a technique that had been piloted in three local hospitals. Following the conference, Mark completed his TRAMm Tracker, indicating only that he had received a certificate as a record of attendance. Six months on, he believes that several service users could benefit from this new practice. He reads further about it, then approaches his team manager, who asks him to plan a strategy for its implementation (including criteria for use). Mark is aware that he has few entries under 'measurement' in his TRAMm Tracker so they discuss ways of rectifying this during supervision.

Case study: Sally revisits TRAMmCPD

In previous chapters we have introduced Sally who has already started to think differently about CPD and how to make the most of learning opportunities. She has explored her strengths and preferred learning style and realises that she needs to be proactive and more strategic in her approach to CPD. After hearing about TRAMmCPD from a colleague and participating in a journal club about CPD engagement, she has visited the TRAMmCPD website and purchased the book about the TRAMm Model.

After downloading the free TRAMmCPD information, TRAMm Tracker and TRAMm Trail (www.TRAMmCPD.com) she has decided to use them to plan and structure her CPD and portfolio. She has read the overview of information about the TRAMm model on the website; and, from her strengths and learning styles preferences (explored in Chapter 4), she knows that she has to do more than just read the information in order to understand it thoroughly. She thinks about the conference she recently attended and links what she did there to the five stations of the TRAMm model. She decides she has visited every TRAMm station, with the following justification:

- **T** (Tell) – yes, she talked to her friends
- **R** (Record) – yes, she used the TRAMm Tracker in the workshop
- **A** (Apply) – yes, she applied it in her portfolio

- **M** (Monitor) – yes, she intends to discuss what she learnt in her next supervision
- **m** (measure) – yes, her CPD certificate is evidence of her attendance at the conference.

    She discusses this with her colleague, who questions whether Sally can really justify her reasoning.

    Read on to Chapter 6 to find out more about how Sally should use TRAMmCPD to reflect what she has done more accurately.

Tasks

The following tasks encourage you to evaluate Sally's use of TRAMmCPD and identify your own learning needs to allow full engagement in the CPD process. You will find it useful to refer to your identified learning needs in order to develop a full profile, which will meet your CPD requirements as the chapters progress.

Is Sally's TRAMm Tracker a good example? To help you answer this question consider the following:

1. Do you think Sally has made effective use of the TRAMm Tracker?
2. Do you agree with the information she has entered? Has she really met HCPC standards 1–4 and visited every TRAMm station?
3. Would you have included anything else?
4. What would you do differently?

Now consider the following questions regarding your own CPD:

5. What is your current approach to CPD? Which (if any) of the examples in this chapter do you identify with?
6. Considering your current approach to CPD, as identified in the previous question, think how the TRAMm Model could help you become more strategic.
7. If you would like to follow Sally's example, go to www.TRAMmCPD.com, download the TRAMmCPD information and record the details of your most recent CPD activities on a TRAMm Tracker.
8. If you have not already done so, read Chapter 4 to identify your strengths and preferred learning style in order to help you identify the strategies that will be most effective for you.
9. Now read Chapter 6 to learn more about how to plan and disseminate your learning (TRAMm station Tell).

A Strategic Guide to Continuing Professional Development for Health and Care Professionals:
THE TRAMm Model

Figure 5.2 TRAMm Tracker: Sally's first attempt at completing a TRAMm Tracker
NB: This does not reflect Sally's CPD (see Chapters 6–10 for more information).

TRAMm Tracker

NAME: Sally OT

Date	Activity description	TRAMm Trail	Reflection	Certificate	HCPC Standards					TRAMm					Index	Notes
					1	2	3	4	5	T	R	A	M	m		
DD/MM/YY	Attended 2 day conference			C	1	2	3	4		T	R	A	M	m	1	Viewed poster display, exhibition, attended sessions: CPD certificate in CPD file

6

How do you plan and disseminate your CPD?
TRAMm Station T: TELL

This chapter explains two essential aspects of communication in relation to CPD and is therefore presented in two parts: Planning and Dissemination. Part 1 defines what we mean by planning, discusses how to plan, and how to use supervision and appraisal/professional development reviews to help identify your CPD requirements. It advises you how to choose the most appropriate types of learning activities and how to articulate those needs.

Part 2, Dissemination, highlights the importance of sharing the outcomes of your CPD and explores the ways in which this can be done. It demonstrates how to make the most of both written and verbal dissemination (including publication, presentation and workshops) with emphasis on how these can be designed and executed with few resources.

Tasks at the end of the chapter will encourage you to consider the potential output from your CPD, linked to your learning needs (as identified following Chapter 3) and the strategic direction of your organisation.

What do we mean by 'Tell' and why is it important?

Talking to others is an essential part of CPD – not only to discuss your own activities and future plans (planning), but also to learn of others' thoughts and ideas and inform them about the activities/outcomes of your CPD (dissemination). The HCPC (2017a, 2019c) and Broughton and Harris (2019) highlight the importance of discussions, interactions and reflecting with colleagues as valid CPD activities and this is supported by Alsop (2013) who, in her book on CPD, dedicates a whole chapter to ways of learning with others and reasons for doing so. The influence of other people, workplace culture and communication are key to the recognition of, engagement in and application of CPD (Lawson 2018).

Talking to others can provide an active forum for learning and help to keep you and others motivated. Alsop (2013) also emphasises the importance of having a sense of belonging and contributing to the whole organisation or community. This adds value to learning, thus providing greater satisfaction. Developing your own learning community can enhance your CPD through professional socialisation and is particularly important if you are a lone worker for instance, in private practice, the only member of your profession within a wider multidisciplinary team (MDT), or you feel unsupported within your team (Lawson 2018, Lawson & Tempest 2019). There are various ways to build your own learning community, some of which are explored throughout this book. These include using social media, developing journal clubs and accessing the support available from your own professional body.

It is important to note that 'Telling' is not only a verbal activity. Much dissemination makes use of the written, rather than the spoken, word – for example, through writing for publication, use of social media and providing project reports. Even in planning we use the written word to articulate our planned activities through setting aims, objectives or goals and recording reflections. Lloyd, Pfeiffer, et al. (2014) found that a key enabler for workplace learning is having access to peers and 'learning networks', again suggesting the importance of communication in CPD.

Part 1: Planning

This first part of the chapter will explore potential communication channels and how they can be used to help you plan your CPD journey.

'Tell' and planning

Please don't assume that 'planning' only means that we expect you to sit and meticulously plan and document your goals/objectives/CPD journey to the very last detail. Although planning can take place in a variety of ways, the more effective you are at planning, the more strategic you become in your approach to CPD. In a study to assess the impact of CPD of Doctors in Primary Care, Mathers, Mitchell & Hunn (2012) found that if CPD was unplanned and not linked to appraisals or organisational objectives, or took place in isolation, there was less chance of it being implemented in practice. As we know, implementation and application in practice are vitally important and therefore classed as mandatory components of CPD according to the HCPC (2017a).

Planning may be formal or informal and some of the things we do often involve planning even though we are unaware we are doing it. Part of the skill is becoming consciously aware of when planning is taking place; once this is clear, future planning skills can be developed or honed. Planning can include:

- Thinking about or articulating what you want to achieve in the next week or month
- Considering what you wish to achieve in the next year or the next 5–10 years
- Thinking about how you might achieve your goals and by when

- Giving opportunities full consideration when they arise
- Identifying clearly articulated SMART (Specific, Measurable, Achievable, Realistic, Timely) aims and objectives.

Whatever your approach to learning and working, it is also important to be flexible in your approach to planning. In Chapter 5 we outlined four different learning/working styles that people recognise in themselves: the ostrich, the bull in a china shop, the procrastinator and the strategist. Some planning is better than none at all; and, as a starting point, planning for each of these approaches may be quite straightforward.

Examples of early stage planning

The ostrich

If you consider yourself to be 'an ostrich' your first goal might be to remove your head from the sand and access www.TRAMmCPD.com to remind yourself of the HCPC standards for CPD. You may also decide to download a TRAMm Tracker and TRAMm Trail, which may be as far as your initial plans go. At this point, you may still have no idea where your CPD is heading. Your next move might be deciding to discuss your lack of direction in your next supervision to clarify your thoughts and help you to explore possible options. You may also talk to some of your more organised peers to ask how they are approaching CPD and find out whether any of their ideas appeal.

The bull in a china shop

You may think yourself more like the bull in the china shop if you say yes to every possible CPD opportunity that presents itself. If this is you, your immediate goal maybe to stand back and take stock of the relevance of each of your CPD activities and identify those that are most appropriate for your current role. At your next appraisal, agree with your line manager your core goals for the forthcoming year only; and any activities you choose will relate to these goals. You may find a TRAMm Tracker useful to begin to index your CPD file, incorporating only the most relevant CPD you have undertaken.

The procrastinator (sitting on the fence)

If you are more of a procrastinator, you may find it difficult to make decisions and perhaps have a tendency to put things off until another day. Your plan will be to stop thinking and start doing. You could start by making a decision to use TRAMmCPD and agree one realistic goal with your line manager that you will be able to achieve by your next supervision.

The strategist

If you are a strategist, you are already well organised, with clear objectives identified and documented in an appraisal or supervision log. This handbook will have been a considered purchase to enable you to further develop your skills using TRAMmCPD as a framework for your professional development.

Informal and formal planning

Planning can be undertaken in a number of ways but, particularly during the early stages of your career, talking to another person can enable you to articulate your thoughts and hear them reflected back, with or without advice on how to pursue your goals. This 'talking' can take place in both informal and formal situations.

Informal planning discussions

These are activities that may be formal or informal in nature but are not specifically designed to enable you to articulate your learning needs. Nevertheless, they may facilitate this by their very nature. Examples of informal discussion opportunities include:

- Talking with peers over coffee
- Networking with other professionals
- Discussion during staff meetings
- Peer group support
- Journal clubs.

A journal club, for instance, is designed for a group of people to discuss and critique new approaches to intervention. However, the subject of learning needs for individuals or the whole department might arise, as can be seen in Example 6.1 below.

Example 6.1 Sanjeev (informal planning discussion)

Sanjeev, an art therapist, decided to coordinate a journal club for his colleagues within a community mental health team. As a team, they are considering integrating co-production as part of their team philosophy. Each team member has been asked to identify one article that explores the effectiveness of co-production in a mental health setting. Following a discussion about the benefits of this for the team and the service users, Sanjeev has been asked how this might fit with his role as an art therapist. He realises that, due to a lack of understanding of co-production, he has not fully considered this. He has now identified this as one of his learning needs so that he can present it to the team in two months' time.

It is important not to underestimate such informal approaches, which provide an invaluable opportunity to air and debate your thoughts in a relatively unconstrained and therefore potentially more creative manner. To illustrate this, it may be useful to consider the most informal discussions you have had – for example, over coffee or lunch with colleagues, which may have prompted new learning opportunities or resolution of clinical dilemmas without attending a conference, course or supervision with a line manager.

Formal planning discussions

Formal mechanisms are those that are specifically designed for you to discuss progress and agree learning needs. They include appraisals or professional development reviews, and the use of supervision or mentorship. (Supervision and Mentorship are discussed in more depth in Chapter 9.)

Example 4.2 Sanjeev (formal planning discussion)

Sanjeev has weekly supervision as part of a comprehensive staff development programme within his community mental health team. At his most recent supervision, Sanjeev discusses his anxieties about the unit's plans to introduce co-production. His manager explores the core reasons for these concerns with him and two issues emerge: he is worried that this will not fit with his role as an art therapist; and he has no other art therapist in the team to discuss this with. At the end of supervision, he agrees two goals with his supervisor, to be completed by the forthcoming week:

1. To find at least one article that comprehensively explores the concept of co-production and its implementation in a community mental health setting

2. To contact his professional body to see whether there are any other art therapists working within a setting that has adopted co-production.

Sanjeev and his supervisor decide that this will be the focus of their discussion the following week. In preparation, Sanjeev has agreed to prepare a summary of what he sees to be the key points about co-production, following his reading of the article. He also decides to reflect on how he sees co-production fitting with his role and where he thinks it may conflict with his role.

Considerations when planning

You may need to consider several issues if your CPD planning is to be effective. These include issues relating to yourself, to the organisation in which you work, what resources are available to you, and possible fallback positions. *The Principles of CPD and Lifelong Learning* (Broughton & Harris 2019) may help to guide you and these aspects are discussed in more detail below.

Issues to consider in relation to yourself

In order to discuss your CPD learning needs and the reasons for these in an informed way, it is important to consider your baseline as a measurement of CPD. This is becoming increasingly important (see Chapter 10), especially when trying to make a case for funding or support towards your CPD activities. This baseline can be mapped by thinking about where you currently are in your career, and the steps you have already taken to get there.

We recommend that you ask yourself the following questions:
- Are your plans realistic?
- Where are you now in your career?

- What skills and knowledge do you have? What have you already achieved?
- What skills and knowledge would you like to have? What would you like to achieve?
- Where do you see yourself in five years' time? What steps do you need to take to help you get there?
- What are your preferred learning styles?
- Which learning styles are you less comfortable with?
- What is the most appropriate way to address your learning needs, taking all these points into account?

You may also find there is a learning and development framework available (see Table 3.1) which may help you to address some of these questions.

Example 6.3 Sanjeev's personal learning needs

Sanjeev has been a qualified art therapist for two years and has spent his time since qualification working for the community mental health team, where he has built up considerable experience using art as therapy when working with people with anxiety and depression. This has given him a clear insight into the factors that can motivate or inhibit recovery.

He has already undertaken one small project in the workplace, which demonstrated the value of art as a means of expression with this group. He feels he now has a general idea of the core principles of co-production but is yet to fully reflect on how this relates to his role and the contribution he can make. He feels this is important, as he would like to remain a valued member of the team should they decide to move forward with this way of working. He is also aware that he is the only art therapist employed in this area who has experience of co-production and is keen that this should become an area of expertise for him. This would help with his future plans to travel abroad to work in an international community.

Sanjeev considers himself to be an auditory learner, who is generally reflective in his approach. He would therefore prefer opportunities that allow him to discuss and reflect upon the implications of the issues explored. He also realises that part of his role will be to work as an activist if the co-production concept is adopted. Following discussion with his manager, he would therefore like to find out more about how he can help drive the implementation forward.

Issues to consider in relation to the organisation in which you work

Having considered your own CPD learning needs, it is also essential to consider those of the organisation for which you work. This is particularly important if you are hoping to use resources from your workplace to enable you to grow and develop. To help you with this, consider the following questions:

- What are the aims of the organisation in which you work now?
- What are their priorities?

- What is their attitude to CPD?
- Who is available for advice and support? If you don't know, how are you going to find out?
- Who do you need to approach to make your case for CPD?

Example 6.4 Sanjeev's workplace organisational priorities

It has been established that Sanjeev's organisation is keen to provide a mental health service that reflects the core principles of a recovery model, and respects the rights and opinions of service users in relation to their own rehabilitation. Despite this innovative outlook, there is no extra government funding available to support this co-production initiative. Sanjeev knows from the organisation's CPD policy that any professional development requirements will need to be supported by a good case, together with an indication of how any additional training may benefit the service and be supported financially.

Mindful that he will need to present his case to the Director of Therapies, he investigates a variety of funding opportunities outside the organisation and identifies a couple of organisations that are already applying this model. Sanjeev contacts two of the organisations for initial discussions to find out how co-production works in practice.

Issues to consider in relation to the resources available to you

Once you have considered yourself and your organisation, you can begin to think about the types of resources at your disposal and how to make the best use of them. These resources are not always immediately obvious, and you may need to be creative in your thinking to maximise your options. This is where talking to others can be particularly useful. Issues to consider include:

- What financial resources are available to you within the organisation?
- What other resources are at your disposal? Who else can assist you?
- What other resources might you be able to utilise that are not immediately obvious?
- How much are you prepared to contribute yourself – in terms of time, money and effort?
- Who do you need to discuss and share your plans with?
- What types of activities are available to address your learning needs, and which are the most appropriate?

If your CPD has been supported by your manager/organisation, it is also important to consider sharing and disseminating the impact of your learning and development with them. Evidence suggests that managers and organisations see little benefit in supporting staff CPD when they do not have tangible evidence of the benefits to the organisation and service users (Haywood, Pain, et al. 2012, 2013). Part of your responsibility may be to make the link between your CPD and the impact on yourself and other stakeholders explicit to encourage future support for CPD – hence the importance of visiting all the TRAMm Stations (Lawson 2018, Lawson & Hearle 2019).

Example 6.5 Sanjeev talks to his colleagues to identify additional resources

Following initial discussions with the Director of Therapies, Sanjeev has established that there is a small staff development fund that provides limited funding for these purposes. There is no specific per capita allocation for each staff member so he is likely to have to compete for funding with other clinical staff in his team. As a member of a specialist mental health interest group, he is also entitled to apply for a small grant towards project development. The local co-production network offers regular free seminars, where people who have adopted this approach are encouraged to disseminate their successes and challenges.

Talking to his immediate colleagues, he realises that they are all in the same situation – all equally keen to develop their understanding of co-production and how it fits with their roles. As a team, they decide to pool their ideas and potential funding sources. They organise a co-production conference, inviting local experts and including service users. They agree that the best way to fund the event is to invite colleagues in other organisations and charge them a small conference fee. This will also provide a good collaborative approach, while allowing opportunities for Sanjeev to discuss his potential role with fellow art therapists in the region.

Sanjeev attends the evening co-production seminars in his own time and at his own expense. The Director of Therapies has agreed that the organisation of the conference can take place in work time as long as clinical caseload continues to be given priority. Sanjeev and his occupational therapy and mental health nurse colleagues agree to share this responsibility.

Issues to consider if the situation changes or your plans change

Although the first part of this chapter has emphasised the importance of plans and discussing these with others, this does not mean that plans are rigid and cannot be changed or amended. On the contrary, it is rare that plans do not change over time – for example, as a result of a change of clinical interest, change of job, change of manager, or change of life circumstances/unforeseen circumstances.

It is essential that alterations to your plans are not viewed negatively but instead seen as a positive opportunity to renegotiate your personal or professional direction. Sailing provides a good analogy for this. Initially, we plot a course to sail to a predetermined destination. We have taken into consideration the wind direction, tide, weather and leeway. Occasionally, due to a sudden, unpredictable change in wind direction, we have to steer to another course. At other times, we may review our journey's progress and decide we need to drop anchor for a while to consider how far we have come, enjoy our current position or even review the course we have planned to follow. Or we may decide to change our intended destination altogether, as a result of choice or necessity. None of these changes is wrong. Each decision is based on a series of carefully considered options, some of which may have resulted from intended or unintended circumstances.

If the situation or your plans change, or you simply change your mind, ask yourself:

- What has caused my plans to change? Is it me and my wishes/life events? Is it the people I work with? Is it the specialist/clinical area I am in? Is it the organisation?
- Is this situation temporary? (You may not want to make drastic changes to your plans if the issue causing you to rethink them is not permanent.)
- What possibilities are now open to me?
- What are the advantages and disadvantages?
- Where do I want to go now?
- What am I going to do next and how?
- Before I change my plans, who can I talk to for advice?
- What are my new goals?

Part 2: Disseminating

'Tell' and disseminating

There are various ways to disseminate the results of your CPD, the choice of which will depend largely on the type of information you want to disseminate, who your audience will be and for what purpose. Again, dissemination can be done informally or formally.

Informal dissemination

Informal mechanisms of dissemination usually happen on an ad hoc basis, with limited planning, forethought or structure. Examples can include:

- Office-based discussion
- Talking in the staff room/socialising
- Internal communication such as email
- Networking
- Social media.

The advantages of these types of communication are that they can relay information immediately and the subsequent discussion may often clarify or change ideas. The disadvantages may be that not everyone gets to know what is being discussed and this can lead to speculation or miscommunication of information. Another disadvantage is that informal discussions are often not recorded, and important information can be missed. This is where the TRAMm Trail can be useful to record brief details, including dates of informal discussions, and who they were with (see Chapter 7).

Although these are informal, mostly unplanned discussions, you still need to think about what you are saying and respect those you are communicating with. You must remain professional in your discussions/correspondence at all times; there are usually consequences for breaking protocols or procedures, even on an informal level.

Formal dissemination

Formal dissemination is that which has been strategically planned in some way. This often involves either written documentation or pre-organised feedback/presentation sessions where you need to send in an application beforehand or be invited by the organisers. The more formal arenas for disseminating your CPD include:

- Conferences/presentations
- In-service workshops/courses/roadshows
- Team exercises/away-days
- Peer-reviewed articles/books
- Projects/pilot studies/service developments reports
- Conference calls
- Social media
- Internal communication (such as intranet, email, staff newsletter)
- Team/preparatory/management meetings
- Supervision/annual appraisal.

Presenting at conferences

Conferences are a popular forum for formally disseminating work undertaken as part of CPD, including work innovations, research and project/service development. There are many important considerations to ensure that you select the most appropriate forum to disseminate your work.

Firstly, consider which type of conference you are going to submit an abstract for; this will largely depend upon your target audience. Conferences are run by a variety of organisations, which may include your professional or regulatory body, your own organisation, private companies, major exhibitions, volunteer committees, and international or European networks. It is important to remember that the activity of presenting at a conference does not, in itself, meet all the HCPC standards. By using TRAMmCPD as a framework for your CPD, you will be able to identify areas that require further consideration.

The work you are presenting may meet HCPC standards 1–4 but the act of presenting the work may only meet standards 1 and 2. The types of things that you might do at a conference to formally disseminate your CPD include:

- Giving a keynote lecture

- Giving a presentation or presenting a paper
- Presenting a poster or a facilitated poster
- Giving an innovative technology presentation
- Running a workshop, seminar or round table discussion.

Giving a keynote lecture

As a keynote speaker, you are generally invited to present an aspect of your work for which you are renowned – either at a national or international level. Being an invited speaker is usually considered an honour, particularly at the larger external conferences. For this, you do not need to propose an abstract but will be expected to provide a short biography, an outline of your presentation and sometimes a copy of your speech for later publication.

Giving a presentation or presenting a paper

Presentations allow you to present information in front of a much larger audience than other types of forum. Timings vary enormously, depending on the particular conference, but the average duration is between 20 and 60 minutes, unless you are presenting a paper.

Presenting a paper gives you an opportunity to present a very concise account of your work. Paper presentations are usually included as part of a themed session containing a further three or four papers on similar subjects and supported by a chairperson to guide the session. Usually a period of approximately 10–15 minutes is allocated for each uninterrupted presentation, plus a further 5 minutes for questions. Questions can either be asked at the end of each presentation or saved until a short panel question-and-answer session, following all presentations in the group. In paper sessions, timing is usually very strict and you will be stopped by the chairperson if you go over your time. It is therefore extremely important to practise your presentation a few times to time it accurately – unless you already have expertise in this area. Copies of your slides, or the reference for a published directly related article, can be made available electronically or via hard copy. If you choose a paper presentation session, you:

- Have a good way of introducing your work to a large audience in a concise manner
- Should expect to benefit from a few (mostly) constructive thoughts on your work, which will provide you with ideas to think about after the conference
- Have the opportunity to meet other interested people at the end of the paper session for further discussion or exchange of contact details.

Presenting a poster or facilitated poster

Within health and social care, as well as in commercial settings and other spheres of life, posters have an important role in informing and educating people. They have also become a popular alternative to presenting papers at conferences. If you also provide an A4 copy of the poster for delegates to take away with them, people can think about the material and contact you at a later date. Facilitated posters provide an opportunity for you to present (usually for about 5 minutes) and discuss your poster with a small group of delegates and fellow poster presenters. Posters have many advantages. They:

- Reach a large number of people
- Can be placed in a wide variety of settings
- Can be used over a long timespan
- Allow the reader to consider material at their own pace
- Provide information using images and clear phrases
- Give information in a non-invasive manner (no stigma)
- Should convey information in an attractive, eye-catching fashion
- Allow for creativity in structuring information
- Allow readers to question and discuss the content if the exhibitor is present.

Giving an innovative technology presentation

If you have designed and produced equipment, software, training materials, videos or communication aids, this gives you a chance to showcase and share these innovations with fellow professionals and obtain immediate feedback. If you choose this option, conference organisers should provide you with space to enable you to provide demonstrations, present a video, or show the product in question. A small visual display area is usually available, along with a tabletop area for you to demonstrate your ideas, although you will usually need to provide your own equipment. The benefits of innovative technology presentations are that they:

- Provide an ideal forum to showcase your innovation in front of a relatively captive audience
- Provide an opportunity for people to see how the innovation should work, possibly try it for themselves and also to ask questions.

Running a workshop

These enable you to pass on your skills to others. Each workshop usually lasts for around 90 minutes and is limited to approximately 20–30 participants. Workshops may be related to practice, management, theory, education or research and development. Ideally, you need to allow time for some 'practical' work, such as practising a skill, discussion groups and trying out tools. You will usually be responsible for chairing and facilitating the session. The benefits of workshops are that they:

- Provide time for skill practice and development
- Allow time for questions and clarification
- Allow a much greater amount of time for discussion and explanation
- Are usually attended by like-minded people to allow exploration of ideas
- Provide an opportunity for people to trial and critique your work.

Running a round table discussion

An interactive discussion (maximum usually approximately 20–30 participants), which enables you to present topics for interactive debate with delegates. Round table discussion sessions usually last for approximately 45–60 minutes, giving plenty of time to debate the topics and get input from delegates working in similar areas. You will usually be responsible for chairing and facilitating these sessions. Although most of the session will be based around audience participation, its success will depend largely upon the trigger used and facilitation of discussion so it is important to give careful consideration to this and engage a co-facilitator if you think this is not your strength. Round table discussions are a good choice if you:

- Have an interest in a hot topic that requires further discussion and debate
- Would like to generate a consensus opinion from a group of colleagues
- Require a short period of focused discussion time with other interested people.

Running a seminar

Seminars are presenter-led sessions, where you have the opportunity to present your topic and allow questions to be raised within the session time. You will usually be responsible for chairing and facilitating the 40–60 minute session, which is based on a certain amount of audience participation but usually less than a round table discussion or workshop. A seminar is a good option to choose if you are looking for a forum that:

- Offers time to present your work in more detail than during a paper presentation
- Allows participants to question and clarify key issues and principles
- Provides an opportunity for you to canvas general opinion.

Applying to a conference

When you are writing and submitting an abstract for a conference, you should consider the following:

- The subject of your abstract.
- Whether to submit it with someone else.
- The target audience.
- Review the overall theme of your work and select the most appropriate conference.
- Alternatively, find out the theme of your selected conference and write your abstract accordingly.
- Note the date and venue in your diary. If you submit an abstract, they will expect you to attend and present.
- Consider where you plan to get funding from (to pay for transport, accommodation and registration) or do you intend to fund your attendance yourself?
- Ethical approval evidence is necessary for all research so ensure that you have this readily available.
- The most appropriate format for your presentation.

When you write the initial abstract, it is wise to complete all the relevant information in a Word document, following the headings and word count instructions. Then you can cut and paste the final information directly into the electronic submission system, ensuring that you have first spell-checked the information and checked it through carefully. As you are writing, it is important to:

- Remind yourself of the conference theme
- Read and ensure that you adhere to the conference guidelines for submitting an abstract, making a note of submission procedures, deadlines and acceptance notification dates.
- Provide a clear title and concise list of contents that meets abstract guidelines
- Ensure you have correctly referenced your abstract, in terms of style and numbers
- Ask someone to check it
- Include a brief biography, if required.
- Before you submit, check all the information has uploaded correctly and print a copy for your records.

Preparing for a conference

Once your abstract has been accepted and you are preparing for the conference:

- Ensure that you adhere to your abstract and the timings. Have you covered everything you have said you will, in the way you have stated you will? For example, if you are presenting a paper, remember it is just that.
- Ask someone to proofread your presentation or poster to eliminate any errors.
- Consider what you will do if the technology fails on the day. What is your back-up plan?
- If you are presenting a poster, how will you get it printed?
- Consider the layout of the room you have been allocated for your presentation.
- Are you going to provide handouts?
- Are you going to have an attendance sheet?
- Will you encourage audience participation and questions throughout, or ask them to wait till the end?
- How does the technology work? You may need to get there early to set the room up as you want, if appropriate.

Tips for audiovisual aids

- You only need the equivalent of four to five bullet points on each slide (prompts only)
- Use cue cards if required
- Practise running through the slides

- Use a combination of relevant pictures and text
- Be consistent in style
- Avoid the use of inappropriate material and take care with cartoons
- Ensure that you (or someone else) check your slides or poster
- Reference your material appropriately and adhere to copyright legislation
- Ensure that the material on the slides is clearly linked to what you are saying.

Tips – verbal skills
- Speak clearly
- Project your voice
- Practise your presentation
- Ensure that you can pronounce all words/names
- Do not make it too complicated
- Use a microphone if one is available
- Do not waffle; be clear and to the point
- If there is something you do not understand, leave it out. Don't try to be clever.

Tips – non-verbal skills
- Stand up
- Check where you are in relation to what you want the audience to be looking at
- Look at the audience or at the back of the room
- Don't wear anything distracting or have anything in your pockets.

Pitfalls – audiovisual aids
- Too much text on the slides or poster
- Slides too busy or too many effects
- Spelling and grammatical errors
- Plagiarism
- Visual material not clearly related to the verbal presentation.

Pitfalls – verbal skills
- Speaking too fast or too slow
- Speaking in a monotone
- Mumbling or speaking too quietly
- Reading from the slides or from sheets of paper
- Being unable to pronounce key words or names.

Other pitfalls
- Poor timing – making your presentation too short or too long
- Not knowing how to use any props
- Using inappropriate material for the target audience
- Having a poor flow in your material
- Trying to be too clever with your information
- Making things up when you don't really know the answer.

And finally
You know more than anyone about what you are presenting but…
- You may not know everything about the subject – others might know more than you
- Be prepared to accept constructive ideas and suggestions and learn from them
- Have a few phrases ready for those who may challenge you aggressively – for example, 'that's a very interesting idea, perhaps we can discuss it further after the presentation'.

Writing for publication

The written word can be a powerful way of disseminating information and allows you to reach a much wider audience than some of the spoken formats highlighted earlier. Written material can be available for reference at a time that is convenient for the reader and has more chance of being cited accurately (although when reading documents, articles or books, it is always important to scrutinise the material with a critical eye). However, the main disadvantage is that written material can often be out of date by the time it is published, particularly if peer review is involved. Information can often take 18–24 months from initial thought to publication and sometimes takes even longer. This delay is partly due to the peer review process, but journals often have themed editions so the editor may hold your article back until the most appropriate edition.

When writing for publication, as with conferences, it is important to think about your target audience. There are a vast range of journals and publishers and careful consideration is required in order to reach the people who are likely to be interested and can make best use of the information. If you decide that the CPD information you have to impart is best suited to a text, identify a range of relevant publishers and look online to see what kind of texts they publish.

When considering other media, you should aim to get your work published in peer-reviewed journals if possible, as these generally reach a wider readership and are considered more credible. If you think a journal may be more appropriate, then it may be useful to visit your organisation's library (or if you have no library, visit the local university or public library) to explore the range of journals available that reflect your topic and target audience. Bear in mind that there is a hierarchy of journals, which is measured by something called 'the impact factor'. This refers to the level of credibility and the expected number of citations and is particularly useful to consider if you are in education and being entered for research assessment. Select a few of the most relevant journals and then look at the types of articles they include and select one that matches your intended style.

When starting your paper, make sure you read the publication guidelines carefully and have them close at hand at all times. All journals are different and it is especially important to take note of the structure (which varies according to the type of article), word count and referencing style. If you don't follow the guidelines, your paper is very likely to be rejected, or you will be required to address the issues anyway.

Most professional journal editors prefer rigorous, ethically approved research so some material may be more suited to professional news magazines, organisational newsletters or web-based reports. Do not be disheartened if your work is not considered suitable for journal publication. This does not mean that it is not valuable and that people do not want to hear about it. In fact publishing in other documents can be just as useful; you get your message out there in a succinct way and it can be a great way of networking and promoting your expertise to others. Check out your professional news magazine or specialist interest group and see what is published there. If you are unsure whether your topic will be of interest, contact the editor or group chairperson (usually listed at the front of the journal or on the website home page). They will often be happy to have a chat about their requirements.

Social media

If you are interested in using technology, social media enables and encourages social interaction anytime, anywhere, from any device (Playfoot & Hall 2018). Web-based and mobile apps 'enable people to create, engage and share content' (Davies, Regina Deli-Amen, et al. 2012, p. 1). There are many and varied forms of social media which, if used wisely, can be a useful and valuable addition to your CPD. Technology is widening the scope of CPD and encouraging the interaction of groups of people by enabling and encouraging the sharing and dissemination of news, information, ideas, resources and advice. Social media provides free, versatile and accessible platforms for offering support, communicating your thoughts and ideas, and sharing best practice.

Engaging in social media can also provide access to a range of key people such as service users, carers, ministers and NHS executives (Holdsworth, Douglas, et al. 2013). There are opportunities to engage in discussion and critical debate not only with other professionals but with people who access services (Maclean, Jones, et al. 2013, Bodell & Hook 2011). The value of learning and being open to hearing both the negative and positive experiences of service users, self-advocates and people with lived experience can encourage greater reflection and insights into the lives and needs of people who use your services.

Social media can also be used to develop your own learning communities by enabling interactions with others which can help you avoid feelings of isolation, encourage collaboration and knowledge sharing. There is the opportunity to promote greater awareness of your role and impact, build new relationships and connect with individuals and organisations both locally and globally. The HCPC emphasises that building informal, professional networks can play an important role in encouraging reflection and retaining competence, as well as improving practice, which should be encouraged and fostered (HCPC 2015, 2017a, 2019c).

It is important that you remain professional and adhere to the HCPC codes of conduct and guidance, as well as those set down by your professional body and employer organisation at all times, both in your professional and private interactions. Unprofessional social media use can result in a HCPC 'fitness to practice' investigation and hearing.

For more information on social media as a CPD activity, see Chapter 2. For ways to Record your social media activities for evidence, see Chapter 7; and for applying your learning from your social media use, see Chapter 8.

Tips on using social media

- Many formats are free to use.
- Ensure you have read and adhere to the HCPC Guidance on Social Media (HCPC 2017b)
- Read and adhere to your professional body guidance on the use of social media
- Read and adhere to your employing organisation's guidance on the use of social media
- Talk to others who already use social media for advice
- Remain professional in all your online interactions, both professional and personal
- Remember that anything you post will be a permanent record, available for anyone to read; if you are in any doubt, do not post
- Ensure your privacy settings are used appropriately and updated regularly
- Maintain service user confidentiality and anonymity at all times
- Start slowly, and see what others are doing, to get a 'feel' for which formats you are more comfortable with; most sites are happy for you to 'lurk' at first, to understand and follow how others are interacting
- Follow people outside your professional sphere to gain a wider view
- Remember that you cannot believe everything you see on social media; Chapter 8 includes information about judging the credibility of what you read.

Roadshows

Roadshows give you an opportunity to showcase something you have developed or wish to promote in order to generate interest outside your organisation. A roadshow is also an opportunity to get information or feedback. For example, as an educationalist you may be designing a new Masters programme for health professionals; the roadshow will enable you to present your initial ideas to a range of people from different areas and receive feedback to ensure that you are meeting the needs of your potential applicants.

Running in-service training

In-service training is usually undertaken by the organisation's staff, for fellow staff members. It can be an effective way of disseminating feedback from CPD; it is usually free of capital costs and, more importantly, it is a way of giving something back to an organisation which (in some cases) has supported you by giving you time and sometimes funding for CPD. In fact, you may suggest running some in-service training as part of your case for attending the CPD in the first place (see Chapter 2). In-service training can take a variety of forms and may include things like skills workshops, case studies or other general feedback presentations, journal clubs and storytelling sessions. It may be a short lunchtime presentation, a full day, or more. Sometimes in-service training is organised internally for staff of the organisation and non-staff members can attend if they pay a small fee. This may be a way of generating further CPD funds for staff, and can again be a good 'output' to include when you argue the case for your CPD.

Case study: Sally learns to discuss and disseminate her CPD through supervision

In previous chapters we have introduced Sally who has already started to think differently about CPD and how to make the most of learning opportunities. She has explored her strengths and preferred learning style and realises that she needs to be proactive and more strategic in her approach to CPD. After hearing about TRAMmCPD from a colleague and participating in a journal club about CPD engagement, she has visited the TRAMmCPD website and subsequently purchased the book about the TRAMm Model.

The following continues from Chapter 5, after Sally has begun to familiarise herself with TRAMmCPD and initiated a TRAMm Tracker.

Sally attends supervision with her manager (who has not yet heard of TRAMmCPD). Sally takes her first completed TRAMm Tracker (Figure 5.2) to discuss what she learnt at the conference (see Chapter 1, Case study), how she now intends to use TRAMmCPD to record her CPD and identify her future learning needs.

Having looked at Sally's TRAMm Tracker, her manager asks how attending the conference means that Sally has met HCPC standards 1, 2, 3 and 4 and how it has benefited her service users. Sally's manager is unclear about the TRAMm stations and after Sally's explanation asks her to deliver a joint 30-minute presentation about TRAMmCPD with her colleague who attended the TRAMmCPD workshop. They will give their presentation at the next monthly allied health professional team meeting, which will include occupational therapists, physiotherapists, a podiatrist, a speech and language therapist, a dietitian and a social worker.

Sally agrees to carry out the following planned actions before her next supervision:
- Amend her TRAMm Tracker to more accurately reflect her achievements in relation to HCPC standards and TRAMm (see Figure 6.1)
- Present what she has learnt in relation to CPD and TRAMmCPD to her colleagues – she can then provide actual evidence for Station T (Tell)
- Start planning for her rotation into Neurorehabilitation and consider how a TRAMm Trail might help her with this in preparation for her next supervision (see Figure 7.7).

Sally and her colleague agree a time and date to do their TRAMmCPD presentation. Sally emails the authors of TRAMmCPD via the website to ask for additional information and they email a copy of their PowerPoint presentation. She downloads and prints off a TRAMm Tracker and TRAMm Trail for everyone. She then sends an email inviting her colleagues to attend a TRAMmCPD lunchtime presentation. After this it is suggested that those who are interested agree to meet every 2 months for a lunchtime CPD meeting, which will alternate with the journal club meetings.

Tasks

The following tasks encourage you to consider the potential outcome from your CPD, linked to the learning needs you identified in Chapter 4 and the strategic direction of your organisation. You should also think about how all these aspects might be linked to each other.

1. Think about your most recent piece of CPD. How could you disseminate the information to your colleagues or other people in your organisation?

2. In your next supervision, can you arrange to discuss your plans? If you do not have a supervision process in your workplace, how can you ensure that you have someone to talk through your CPD plans with? Do you need to set one up?

3. If you have not already done so, download a TRAMm Tracker from www.TRAMmCPD.com and begin to record your most recent pieces of CPD.

4. Initiate a TRAMm Trail (free to download from www.TRAMmCPD.com) for your most significant piece of recent CPD and focus your attention on Station T for that specific CPD activity. If you have nothing to record in this section, think about what you can do to rectify this. Remember to record the dates and to continue to update your TRAMm Trail (see Chapter 7 for details about what to include).

5. Do you agree with the information Sally has recorded in her TRAMm Tracker? Would you have recorded something different? Why?

6. Has any of your CPD had a tangible, measurable impact on yourself, your team, your service users and/or your organisation? If so, how can you share this positive impact to encourage support for your future CPD plans?

7. Read on to Chapter 7 to learn more about ways of recording your CPD (TRAMm station R – 'Record').

Figure 6.1 Sally's amended TRAMm Tracker (entries in blue are updates from previous chapter)

Date	Activity description	Certificate	Reflection	TRAMm Trail	1	2	3	4	5	T	R	A	M	m	Index	Notes
DD/MM/YY	Introduced to TRAMmCPD by a colleague in a staff meeting				1	2				T	R	A				Learning about TRAMmCPD organising to present information to colleagues
DD/MM/YY	National Professional Conference Day 2	C			1						R				2	Attended Stroke Rehabilitation Seminar Conference attendance certificate in CPD file
DD/MM/YY	Attended National Professional Conference Day 1	C			1						R				1	Viewed poster display & exhibition Attended Professional Use of Social Media Session – useful information stored in CPD file

7

How do you record your CPD plans and activities?
TRAMm Station R: RECORD

This chapter explores why it is important to record your CPD and the mechanisms by which CPD can be recorded, including personal and professional development plans, learning contracts, reflections/reflective models and portfolios. We will introduce the TRAMm Tracker and TRAMm Trail as potential tools for recording your CPD and completed examples of both are included, to illustrate their use.

Tasks at the end of the chapter will encourage you to consider the most effective ways to record information that reflect your own learning and retrieval styles. A portfolio format will be suggested, and you will be encouraged to complete at least one reflection using a reflective model template and one record using the TRAMm Trail.

What do we mean by 'Record'?

Recording is the process of capturing data in written or other permanent form, for the purpose of preserving evidence (*Oxford Paperback Dictionary and Thesaurus* 2007). There are many different ways to record data, both formal and informal. Suggestions for items you might include in your Station 'R' Record are listed in Table 5.1. Whatever you record for your CPD, you must remember to protect the anonymity of service users and stakeholders, ensuring that anything submitted for HCPC audit or shown to another person remains completely confidential (HCPC 2017c).

Why do we need to record CPD?

It is your responsibility as a professional to initiate, undertake and record your CPD. The HCPC Standard 1 (HCPC 2017a, p.5) states that registrants must maintain a 'continuous, up to date and accurate record of their CPD activities' and 'keep a record of CPD, in whatever format is most convenient'. In addition, the HCPC and all the registered health and care professional bodies provide members with a code of ethics and professional conduct that outlines your responsibility as a registered professional for actively maintaining and continuing your professional development and for retaining a record of your CPD.

From your own perspective, regardless of guidelines, it is an important part of evidencing your development over time and receiving credit for the things you have achieved. It is also intrinsically rewarding to have a record showing that you have made a difference to the lives of service users and students through your professional career.

How and when should we record our CPD?

In Chapter 4 we discussed the uniqueness of each individual in terms of strengths, and preferred working and learning styles, and the same applies to recording CPD. If you are a visual learner, you are likely to prefer recording mechanisms that provide a visual snapshot of your learning, such as the TRAMm Trail, TRAMm Tracker or a mind map. If you are a read/write learner, you may prefer to undertake a written reflection first, and fill in your formal record later, once you have decided what you have learnt.

There are many different ways to record your CPD and it is a question of personal preference whether you use traditional pen and paper or an electronic recording method. Online technology is a popular method, as it is convenient to store, and quick and easy to update as you progress. This form of recording keeps evolving and now includes media such as videos, voice recordings and e-collation methods. Various methods of recording your CPD are explored in more depth below.

Reflective logs

Reflection is the process of analysis, critical awareness and self-evaluation that results in a change of practice. It allows us to learn from our experiences and plays a large part in the development of knowledge and skills (Constable 2013). Chapter 2 highlights how reflection can be undertaken as a CPD activity and Chapters 9 and 10 explore the use of reflection in monitoring and measuring progress. In this chapter, we look at the ways in which we can record our reflections.

There are several formats for keeping reflective logs, including the use of a structured template for supervision, written accounts following a specific reflective model, and the use of social media such as 'blogging' or weblogs.

Reflective logs are exploratory, self-critical accounts of a process or critical event. Their aim is to explore the reasons why something has happened and what influenced the outcome. They can also help you identify how things could be done differently, from both an objective and subjective perspective. This may not only include description and evaluation of the process or event but can also involve exploration of emotive aspects such as your own (or others') feelings, values and attitudes, which may have contributed to the outcome. Reflective logs should always lead to either a change or validation of practice. Any actual changes to practice, together with their impact, can be added to the log at a later date.

Various models can be accessed to facilitate written reflections and the selection of model is very dependent upon personal preference and reflective style. All have similar criteria but they differ in their emphasis and the terminology they use. Examples include:

- Schon (1983): Reflection in and on action
- Gibbs (1988): Reflective cycle, six stages – description, feelings, evaluation, analysis, conclusion and action plan
- Boud (1988): Follows a three-stage process – returning to the experience, attending to the feelings and re-evaluating the experience
- Johns (1994): Nuances of reflection; involves a series of questions that help structure the practitioner's reflections, supervision and keeping of a structured reflective diary; designed as a reflective nursing model but questions can be adapted to other fields
- Fish and Twinn (1997): four strands of reflection – 1. factual strand (what happened); 2. retrospective strand (looking for patterns and meaning); 3. sub-stratum strand (exploring assumptions/values/feelings); and 4. connective strand (implications for practice and plans)
- Rodgers (2002): four-stage reflective cycle – presence, description, analysis and experimentation.
- Rolfe, Freshwater and Jasper, (2001): Follows a three-stage process with three simple questions: What? So what? and Now what?

If you would like to explore any of these models further, references are provided at the end of this book.

Mind maps

Mind maps provide a visual tool with which to organise your thoughts around a subject (see Figure 7.1, page 96). They are a useful way to record a brief summary of your CPD in relation to a specific topic and identify links between relevant areas. They also provide a one-page snapshot that can act as a catalyst for discussion in supervision or mentorship sessions (see Chapter 9). Mind maps usually contain less detail than the TRAMm Trail but a little more than the TRAMm Tracker. They can therefore act as a useful bridge between the two, to act as a reminder of what you have achieved. You can then return to your mind map later, in order to jog your memory for your TRAMm Trail and reflections. There are websites that provide mind map templates, which may be worth exploring in the first instance. Figure 7.1 applies the mind map concept to the content of this chapter.

Learning contracts

Learning contracts are collaboratively written and agreed documents that indicate what will be learnt, the resources to be used, and how the learning will be evaluated and evidenced or validated. They offer a concise way of explicitly recording learning needs in relation to a specific context. These contracts are often used by students on placement, when they have generic learning outcomes specified by their university that need localising to their placement setting.

They can be considered as working documents. During their completion, it must be clear exactly how the learning need will be demonstrated and who will validate each piece of evidence.

A useful template is shown in Table 7.1 (page 97).

A Strategic Guide to Continuing Professional Development for Health and Care Professionals:
THE TRAMm Model

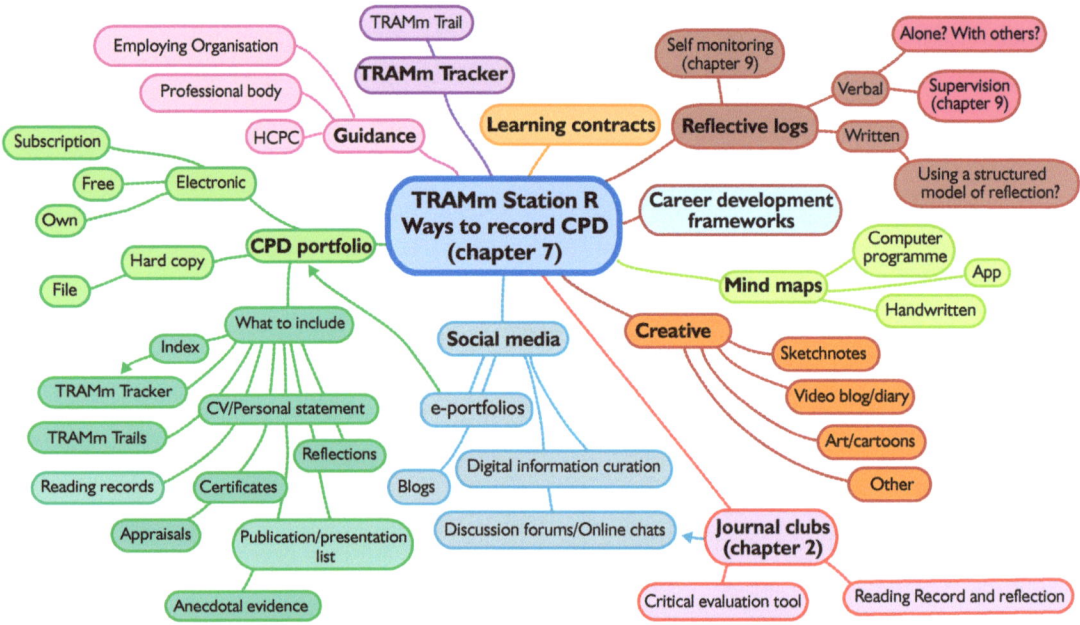

Figure 7.1 Example of a mind map

Compiling portfolios

A portfolio is an organised collection of evidence designed for a specific purpose. In the same way as an artist, photographer or designer produces a portfolio to showcase their ability, we too can develop portfolios that showcase our professional ability through our CPD.

Portfolios are confidential documents, either in hard copy or electronic format, which you can choose to share with others in full or in part. They can be for your own personal use or compiled for a particular purpose (Constable 2013) such as job interviews. When organising your portfolio, you can also have 'public' and 'private' sections, where the private section is easy to remove if necessary. It is important to note that a portfolio is not the same as the profile that you are expected to complete as part of your HCPC audit (see Chapter 10).

These terms are often used interchangeably, but in this book we define them as follows:

- CPD portfolio: your personal evidence of all your CPD engagement; relevant sections can be shared at job interviews, as part of your ongoing appraisal process, and provide a resource for retrospective reflections on your professional progress.
- CPD profile: an overview of your professional highlights, areas of expertise and experience. For example, you would submit your CPD profile if selected for HCPC audit.

Table 7.1 Example of a learning contract template

Learning need (What do you want to learn?)	Resources (What resources can you utilise to help you to learn?)	Evidence (How can you show you have achieved what you set out to learn?)	Validation (Who will confirm your evidence and when?)
1. How to undertake my CPD and what evidence to provide for it	Text: Hearle, Lawson and Morris (2020). *A Strategic Guide to CPD for Health Professionals: The TRAMm Model* TRAMm Tracker TRAMm Trail Colleagues examples	Portfolio format designed by DD/MM/YY Complete relevant sections on the TRAMm Tracker Undertake 1 TRAMm Trail for an element of CPD	Line manager in supervision: …………………… TRAMm mentor via online support: ……………………
2. Models of reflective practice	Internet/databases Search terms: Reflective models Portfolios in healthcare	Two written reflections: One following Gibbs' model of reflection and the other following Boud, by DD/MM/YY	Line manager in supervision: ……………………

You can take various approaches to compiling your professional portfolio, but the important thing to remember is that it should represent you and what you have achieved. It is much better to have one portfolio with content entirely produced by you, rather than three or four enormous files containing leaflets, instructions, reports and articles written by other people, with very little reflection or 'real' evidence of your CPD and how it has influenced your practice and your own and others' performance.

Content to consider including in your CPD portfolio

This is a list of the sort of things you might consider including but it is not exclusive. Remember to anonymise service users or other sensitive information.

Introduction to your CPD and portfolio:
- TRAMm Tracker or another continuous, up-to-date and accurate CPD record
- You may also require an index if you are not using a TRAMm Tracker.

Introduction to you:
- Your Curriculum Vitae

- A personal statement
- List of your publications and presentations (see Chapter 6).

Evidence of your CPD:

- Learning contracts
- Appraisals
- Supervision, preceptorship and/or learning and development records
- TRAMm Trails
- Reflections on your practice/courses/significant incidents
- Other creative reflective work, such as stories, poems or diary excerpts
- Reading record
- Intervention evidence records (see Chapter 8)
- Evidence of additional responsibilities (such as supervision of students) or advanced practice following the four pillars, i.e. practice, management/ leadership, education and research, especially if you are aiming for promotion
- Summaries of research or evaluation reports, alongside a reflection on your contribution to them
- Summaries and reflections on roles within your professional sphere such as professional body activities, external examining and interprofessional roles
- Summaries of roles outside your professional work that you have undertaken (or that you are currently undertaking), together with a critical commentary on their application to your current work. For instance, if you are a tennis coach or a school governor or teach photography in your spare time, this may be relevant.

Other evidence of your CPD:

- Certificates
- Details of any awards, with descriptions of the awards
- Testimonials
- Anecdotal evidence (see Chapter 8).

Organising your CPD portfolio

It is personal preference how you choose to organise your CPD portfolio but you must remember that it needs to be accessible, logically ordered, functional and easy to update. You can design the structure yourself, follow your professional body's guidance or utilise an online portfolio builder. The other way to organise your portfolio is to use TRAMmCPD to provide a framework. A well-structured CPD portfolio enables you to present and access information easily for job or other applications, interviews, discussions at appraisal, HCPC audit and accreditation exercises.

Online CPD portfolios

Online, cloud based, CPD portfolio and management systems from private companies are increasingly available, generally for a monthly subscription fee. These enable you to record and upload documents via a computer and apps on smart devices. If selected for HCPC audit, you can then download and print the information as part of your CPD profile submission. There is mixed evidence available as to the efficacy of such online portfolios. Some authors (Illing, Crampton, et al. 2017, Silversides 2015) suggest that online recording can save time and make the audit process more efficient. However, there is little evidence of explicit consideration of the wider aims of CPD engagement or whether learning is used and applied in practice or whether there are improved service user outcomes (Foucault, Vachon, et al. 2017; Vachon, Foucault, et al. 2018).

As with many other aspects of CPD, support and mentorship from others, and integration of these tools within team and work environments, may encourage greater recognition of and engagement in CPD, as well as the application of learning in practice. Following the stations of the TRAMm Model whilst using these platforms may help to ensure that you are fully engaged in the process of CPD, rather than just storing copies of attendance certificates with no consideration of the wider aims of CPD.

As with all forms of online technology, it is important to ensure that you understand the terms and conditions of use, how secure your data will be, whether the company complies with GDPR (Great Britain 2018), and who they share your data and information with.

See Chapter 2 for more on using social media as a CPD activity; see Chapter 6 for ways to use social media to help plan and disseminate your learning ('Tell'); see Chapter 8 for things to consider when applying learning gained from your use of social media.

Ways to record your online interactions

There are various methods available to record evidence of your online interactions, which may contribute to your CPD. Some of these may be developed and accessed via your professional bodies, others by paid subscription to private companies. Methods such as e-portfolios, digital curation tools, information collation tools and blog platforms are available at little or no cost. They provide an opportunity to document your thoughts, share ideas, store useful information, disseminate information and advertise your role or service. Whichever method you use, you must always exercise caution, check the terms and conditions of use, how your information will be shared and with whom, and follow the guidelines (set out by the HCPC, your professional body, employer and other organisations) regarding the use of social media and online recording.

Weblogs (known as blogs) offer a way to record your personal observations, reflections, opinions and thoughts, which may be shared on a website, and many of them are free to use.

Some sites allow you to keep your blog private or invite selected people to view what you have written or make it freely available to the public. Reading other people's blogs can also give you useful information but, as with all social media, caution is required: they are not peer-reviewed and care must be taken when interpreting or using any information gleaned from them (Moorley & Chinn 2015). For more on weblogs, see Chapter 8.

Online information collation tools enable you to capture, as a transcript, your online conversations and even allow you to make further comments. To fully utilise these tools, some time and skill are required. It may be possible to use links to your collation tool as part of your evidence of CPD. Alternatively, a quicker, simpler option may be to take screenshots of your discussions as proof of your interactions.

If you choose to participate in discussion forums, online chats and/or online journal clubs, record your participation in your TRAMm Tracker, including dates with relevant links. For the most significant sessions and interactions, you could initiate and update a TRAMm Trail, including what you contributed to, where to access the information in the future and how you have used the information you have learnt (see Chapter 8).

For online journal clubs to be most effective as a CPD activity, you should ensure that you select relevant chats in which to participate, critically evaluate the article using an appraisal tool, complete a reading record, and write or record a reflection to show how you will apply what you have learnt (see Chapter 8). You could also consider whether you can disseminate (Tell) what you have learnt to your colleagues and the most effective way to do this (see Chapter 6).

A record of your social media activity may contribute useful evidence for your CPD. Many of the social media activities you have engaged in will be freely available online, and the HCPC may accept links to your social media activity if it is relevant to the CPD profile you are submitting. For major pieces of evidence, it may be worth printing your social media evidence in order to provide the HCPC with copies.

A document by NHS Employers (2016) provides further guidance regarding the use of social media. It is essential to remember that the popular platforms of social media are constantly changing, and it is important to choose your options wisely. You must also ensure that you observe and adhere to all the professional guidance regarding the use of social media and remember that there is no distinction between private and work life when you are a registered health and care professional. Be very careful about what you (or your friends and colleagues) post and ensure that your privacy settings are activated and that you regularly check them.

See Chapter 2 for more on using social media as a CPD activity; see Chapter 6 for ways to use social media to help plan and disseminate your learning ('Tell'); see Chapter 8 for things to consider when applying learning gained from your use of social media.

Using the TRAMm Tracker and TRAMm Trail to record your CPD

TRAMmCPD encompasses the TRAMm Model, TRAMm Tracker and TRAMm Trail. (The TRAMm Model and its development are discussed in Chapter 5.) The TRAMm Tracker and TRAMm Trail have been developed as tools to complement the TRAMm Model and help you engage with and record your CPD (Hearle, Lawson & Morris 2016).

The TRAMm Tracker (see Figure 7.3, p. 111) has been designed as an adaptable tool to record and measure your individual learning outcomes, while taking into account the HCPC standards for CPD. The TRAMm Tracker:

- Allows you to track your progress
- Offers you the opportunity to record, monitor and measure your professional development, as you work towards fulfilling the HCPC registration standards
- Enables you to cross-reference your learning between TRAMm stations
- Helps you identify gaps in your learning needs
- Acts as an index for your CPD portfolio.

The TRAMm Trail (Figure 7.4, p.112) has been designed, following feedback received, to encourage you to plan and record in a little more depth the most significant pieces of your CPD, which you may need to use if you are called for HCPC audit. The TRAMm Trail:

- Enables you to strategically plan your learning and development across the TRAMm stations
- Acts as a brief summary of your work and learning
- Enables you to record more specific details than the TRAMm Tracker
- Can be used alongside your favoured method of reflection.
- Is easy to complete and can be referred to later when completing your reflections.

Feedback from the pilot evaluation suggests that people have found it most effective to use both their TRAMm Tracker and TRAMm Trail as 'works in progress', updating them as they go along. They have also used them in their supervisions and annual appraisals to highlight what has been achieved and identify future learning needs (see Chapters 9 and 10). Some people use a weekly or monthly alarm to remind them to update their TRAMmCPD; this has been referred to by one participant as their own personal TRAMm nagger!

How and when should you use the TRAMm Tracker and TRAMm Trail?

This chapter focuses on the TRAMm Tracker and TRAMm Trail as methods of recording your CPD; Chapter 10 will highlight how they can be used to measure your CPD. The TRAMm Tracker is used to record your engagement in your CPD and can be submitted to the HCPC as your chronological record of your CPD activities (HCPC CPD Standard 1). The TRAMm Trail enables you to record your plans and thoughts about things you intend to do, as well as providing greater depth on things you have already done. The TRAMm Tracker, with relevant TRAMm Trails, can be submitted to the HCPC as part of the evidence for your CPD Profile and we know people who have successfully done this using TRAMmCPD. It should be noted that the HCPC does not endorse any particular tools, or that their use guarantees success if selected for audit. However, they do acknowledge that tools like TRAMmCPD can provide useful ways to structure and record your CPD (HCPC 2017a).

The HCPC information about *How to Complete your Continuing Professional Development Profile* (HCPC 2019d) provides full details of what you are required to submit for audit. At the time of writing, the HCPC are trialling online submission of CPD profiles; more information is available via their website: https://www.hcpc-uk.org

The HCPC does stress that you should use whatever method works for you, that all activities must be dated, in chronological order and that everything you submit must be your own work. It is important to remember these points when using your TRAMm Tracker and TRAMm Trail, as the most common issues in the HCPC audit feedback (2019b) are that registrants fail to supply dates, fail to demonstrate that they are undertaking a mixture of different learning activities, fail to number/label pages, and focus on quantity rather than quality. The HCPC (2019b) advises that you only choose between four and six activities from the last two years to use as evidence. This is useful to remember when reflecting on your CPD. The TRAMm Tracker enables you to identify, at a glance, all your CPD that meets HCPC standards 1–4 and visits all the TRAMm stations. From these, you can choose which activities to provide detailed evidence for, if you are selected for HCPC audit.

To decide what to record in your TRAMm Tracker and TRAMm Trail, it is important to recognise all forms of potential learning. For instance:

1. When you are learning something new which needs to be recorded as CPD and/or when your routine work has developed into CPD (see Chapter 3). This is when you notice that you have stopped working on 'automatic pilot' and you are employing an activity (see Chapter 2) in order to learn something new.

2. When your usual intervention has had an unintended consequence and/or you have been asked to undertake something new, of which you have little or no experience. In this case you may have reflected on the reasons for this and the changes required to your practice as a result.

3. Through supervision or appraisal, you may have identified a new way of working or perhaps you are beginning to develop advanced skills in order to further your career.

4. You may have attended a training event in the past and have recently used the knowledge gained to improve your practice and a service user's outcome.

At any of these points, a new entry or an update to an existing entry in your TRAMm Tracker may be needed. It is entirely up to you when to initiate or update a TRAMm Trail. You may decide you have too much information to record briefly in your TRAMm Tracker or you may recognise that there is significant learning taking place, which needs to be recorded in more depth. It must be stressed that the TRAMm Trail should be used alongside your favoured method of reflection to fully record your learning and outcomes. Mapping your usual work activity into TRAMmCPD could highlight that you are, in fact, developing your practice and your activities have crossed over into CPD. This is then worth recording in more depth.

How to complete your TRAMm Tracker

This is available as a free download from www.TRAMmCPD.com.

As discussed earlier, the decisions about which TRAMm stations each piece of your CPD visits are entirely subjective, although some suggestions are included in the opening sections of Chapters 6–10. The TRAMm Tracker is designed to be used as a working document, to be initiated and added to over time. It is not anticipated that you will necessarily meet each HCPC standard or visit every TRAMm station for every piece of your CPD. Initially, you may only complete HCPC standards 1 and 2 and visit TRAMm station R (Record) but, as time passes and you use what you have learnt, you can revisit and update your TRAMm Tracker. It is important to date every entry, as the HCPC (2017a) asks for explanations if you have gaps of three or more consecutive months which suggests that you aim for at least one CPD activity every two months.

You will see that Figure 7.2 (p. 110) provides an outline of page 1 and a brief overview of the five HCPC standards, along with some suggestions for each of the TRAMm stations. Remember: by keeping an up-to-date TRAMm Tracker, you will be meeting HCPC Standard 1, and Standard 5 is only met if you are called for HCPC audit. Figure 7.3 (p. 111) provides an outline of page 2 of the TRAMm Tracker. You may also note that the sample TRAMm Trackers have the most recent entries at the top of the form; this enables you to quickly add new entries without scrolling through the whole document. However, you are of course entirely free to arrange your TRAMm Tracker as it suits you.

Remember that the Tracker is only designed to provide an 'at-a-glance' index record of all CPD undertaken and achieved, whether formal or informal. Sometimes it can be difficult to decide whether you need to add an additional row in the Tracker or to expand one that is already started. For example, you attend a course on designing the environment for people with dementia and log this on your Tracker. During your work with a service user with dementia, you subsequently realise that you need more information on the types of equipment that would be useful in the bathroom. You therefore contact a colleague in a local dementia unit, who has the required expertise, and arrange a visit. Is this a new CPD activity or a continuation of the original one? The decision is yours, as long as the information is documented. In this situation it is more likely that you would continue with the original Tracker row, as the activities are clearly linked, and it would allow you to visit additional TRAMm stations. Alternatively, you could choose to start a new line and cross-reference the link between the two in the Notes column.

Table 7.2: The TRAMm Tracker: A brief overview

Page/Column	Content
Page 1	Overview of the five HCPC standards, along with suggestions for each of the TRAMm stations.
Page 2	The TRAMm Tracker
Column 1: Date	Date/s when activity/activities took place (state if ongoing)
Column 2: Activity description	Brief title of CPD activity carried out, with brief description of the activity/what you did
Columns 3, 4, 5: Certificate, Reflection and Trail	Record whether you received a Certificate of Attendance, have written/recorded a reflection and/or initiated a TRAMm Trail about the activity
Column 6: HCPC standards	Enter the HCPC standard/s you feel each CPD activity meets. Initially you may only meet Standards 1 and 2. As time passes and you carry out more work/learning, you may revisit your Tracker and complete more standards. It is not expected that every piece of your CPD will meet all HCPC standards. You will find more information in HCPC (2017a) *Continuing Professional Development and Your Registration*.
Column 7: TRAMm stations	Enter the TRAMm station/s you feel you have visited for each CPD activity. Initially you may only visit the 'R' (Record) station. As time passes, and you carry out more work/learning, you may revisit your Tracker and visit more stations. It is not expected that you will visit each station for every activity or piece of CPD (see Chapters 6–10 for more information regarding each station).
Column 8: Index	This column relates to the index within your CPD file/portfolio, where each piece of hard evidence is stored. If your evidence is stored electronically, there is space to record this, or add a link to it in column 10 Notes. There will not always be a need to record anything in this column.
Column 9: Notes	This column is for you to record your own notes on items that you feel are most relevant – for example, your cross- references to workplace competencies which may include KSF standards, learning and development frameworks (see Chapter 3), where you have stored information, where to find other related pieces of evidence, etc.

Some questions you could ask yourself in order to make the decision include:

1. Does this activity link directly to the same learning need as the main row? (If not, start a new row.)
2. Is it a very distinctive new activity, such as a course? (If yes, start a new row.)

3. Have I learnt or done very different things in this new CPD activity? (If yes, start a new row.)

4. Is the Notes column too full and lacking in clarity? (If yes, start a new row or initiate a TRAMm Trail to record more information.)

5. Is what you are trying to record becoming confusing or unwieldy? (If so, initiate TRAMm Trail(s).) You may need to separate out the learning events. For example, Sally's record of conference attendance in Chapter 6 has been separated into conference day 1 and conference day 2.

For significant pieces of CPD, to plan your future learning needs or to provide a reminder, you may wish to record details in a little more depth using the TRAMm Trail or other recording mechanisms such as reflections.

The TRAMm Tracker was originally developed to encourage you to maintain a continuous up-to-date record of your CPD. However, after the twelve-month pilot evaluation feedback, it became apparent that it was difficult to remember why certain columns had been completed. The TRAMm Trail was then developed as a method to plan future development and CPD activities and also as a way to record learning/activities that have taken place in more depth. The 'Plan of Action' section enables registrants to record their future plans, identified from their Tracker and Trail.

The TRAMm Tracker and TRAMm Trail can also be used when preparing for job interviews and annual appraisals by helping you identify the most relevant pieces of CPD and decide which CPD evidence is most pertinent to the job or role for which you are applying.

How to complete your TRAMm Trail

The TRAMm Trail has a dual purpose. It can be used to plan your CPD strategically to achieve your outcome: what it is you want to achieve and how you are going to get there (see Figure 7.5, p. 113). The TRAMm Trail also offers you a method of recording in a little more depth the most significant pieces of your CPD, which you may use if you are called for HCPC audit. The Trail has been designed to provide a brief summary of work and learning, to be used alongside your favoured method of reflection.

The TRAMm Trail has a section for each of the TRAMm Stations (Tell, Record, Apply, Monitor and Measure), together with a 'Plan of Action' section (see Chapters 6–10). You can document as much or as little as you wish, and record it according to your preferred style (such as words, pictures, captions or cartoons) to remind you what you plan to achieve, with timescales, or what you did and when.

Remember, it is vital to include dates and where to find the relevant evidence if required. On some occasions, you may decide that the same piece of evidence or learning needs to be recorded in more than one TRAMm station. For instance, your appraisal might be included in TRAMm 'T' as a discussion of your learning needs, 'R' as a written record, and alongside 'm' as a successful measure of your professional achievements.

Like the TRAMm Tracker, the TRAMm Trail is designed to be used as a 'work in progress' to update regularly and keep as a working document. It can then act as a prompt, alongside your favoured method of reflection. Once completed, the relevant TRAMm Trails can be submitted as evidence if you are called for HCPC audit.

Avoid trying to record too many learning experiences in one TRAMm Trail, as this can become confusing. If this is the case, it may be advisable to break the learning/event down and use more than one Trail.

Example 5.1 India's use of TRAMm Tracker and TRAMm Trail

India (a student dietitian) recorded her eight-week placement, along with the case study she presented to her educators, in one line of her TRAMm Tracker and the details in one TRAMm Trail. She found that her Tracker and Trail became very lengthy and she was becoming confused between what was placement learning and what was specific to the case study. She was advised to break the learning into two separate but linked entries on her TRAMm Tracker and TRAMm Trails, as follows:

- TRAMm Tracker entry/Trail 1 – An overview of the whole placement experience, where she recorded what she had learnt, including brief reference to the case study she presented.
- TRAMm Tracker entry/Trail 2 – Case study: A more detailed record of the learning carried out with the service user, including the assessment, planning, intervention, outcome process and the self-directed informal research she carried out into the medical condition, alongside the skills learnt to use a slideshow presentation programme to present the case study. India also completed a written reflection.

Table 7.3 The TRAMm Trail: A brief overview of sections and suggested content

Section	Suggested content
TRAMm Trail title	Link your title to columns 2 and 3 in your TRAMm Tracker.
Date	Date that you initiated your TRAMm Trail; remember that each entry should include a date where relevant and/or note that work is ongoing.
Tell (T)	Record relevant conversations and discussions, who you discussed your future plans with, disseminated information to etc. (see Chapter 6 for more details).
Record (R)	Record of evidence, when and where the evidence is stored (see Chapter 7 for more details).
Apply (A)	Briefly record how you have ensured the credibility of what you have learnt and how you have used your learning in practice (see Chapter 8 for more details).

Monitor (M)	List how you are monitoring your learning considering constructive feedback or self-critique (see Chapter 9 for more details).
measure (m)	Briefly enter how you are measuring the impact of your CPD on yourself and others, the outcomes achieved that meet the HCPC standards 1–4 and which TRAMm stations (see Chapter 10 for more details).
HCPC standards met	Enter which HCPC standards you believe this piece of CPD meets.
Plan of action	What do you plan/need to do next? As you achieve these aims, they can be moved to the relevant station within your TRAMm Trail and you can update the relevant entry in your TRAMm Tracker.

In your TRAMm Trail, it is likely that you will visit other stations to record your thoughts about what you plan or intend to do. By planning you are engaging in 'T' (Tell) and by working on a Trail you are making an 'R' (Record). As you carry out your plans, undertake your activities, apply your learning and achieve your goals, you can begin to complete more stations within your TRAMm Trail and update your TRAMm Tracker to record what you have achieved.

As an example, consider Sally's TRAMm Tracker (see Figure 7.6, p. 115) and her TRAMm Trail, entitled 'Rotation into neurorehabilitation' (see Figure 7.7, p. 116). In her TRAMm Tracker she has ticked 'T' because she has begun planning for her rotation with her supervisor and 'R' because she has initiated a TRAMm Trail to 'record' her plans. In her TRAMm Trail, however, she has written and recorded her plans in every TRAMm station. The entries in *italic* type are the plans she has made. As she achieves each one, she will remove the italic type and complete the relevant column in her TRAMm Tracker.

Case study: Sally uses TRAMm Tracker and TRAMm Trail to record her CPD

In previous chapters we have introduced Sally who has already started to think differently about CPD and how to make the most of learning opportunities. She has explored her strengths and preferred learning style and realises that she needs to be more proactive and strategic in her approach to CPD.

After hearing about TRAMmCPD from a colleague, and participating in a journal club about CPD engagement, she has visited the TRAMmCPD website and purchased the book about the TRAMm Model. Having familiarised herself with TRAMmCPD and initiated her TRAMm Tracker in Chapter 5, she has started to use TRAMmCPD in supervision to help identify and articulate her CPD plans. In Chapter 6, she began to engage in ways of planning and disseminating her learning.

One of Sally's identified needs during supervision was to start planning for her rotation into neurorehabilitation. In preparation for her next supervision, Sally initiates her first TRAMm Trail, which includes a record of the things she thinks she needs to do towards her forthcoming rotation. With her supervisor, Sally records the outcomes of her supervision, including a set of negotiated and agreed goals, as follows:

1. To contact the senior occupational therapist in neurorehabilitation to ask if there is any preparation that she would like Sally to do.

2. To learn more/recap her neuroscience anatomy knowledge, using publicly available online video learning material, and understand its relevance for practice; to be explained to her supervisor at the next supervision session.

3. To understand the application of neurodevelopmental approaches in preparation for practice. (As Sally is not yet in neurorehabilitation, she is not sure how to make this 'live' but she makes a few notes and decides to take it to a second pre-meeting with her prospective new line manager.)

4. To speak to a Band 5 who is rotating away from neurorehabilitation at the next peer support group; to discuss with other Band 5s what they have done that was useful.

5. To investigate the NICE guidelines and care pathways for Stroke and document the relevant aspects for her role as an occupational therapist.

6. To investigate further training opportunities for neurorehabilitation.

7. To reflect upon her anxieties about rotating into a specialist area and discuss this at her next supervision.

8. To initiate a TRAMm Trail, to record in more detail the work she has done around TRAMmCPD, and to update it as she uses what she has learnt (see Figure 7.8, p. 117).

Following her supervision, Sally updates her TRAMm Tracker to include a reference to presenting TRAMmCPD at the Allied Health Professions meeting. She completes the additional HCPC standards and TRAMm stations she has met and initiates a TRAMm Trail (see Figure 7.7, p. 116) for her forthcoming rotation.

She also records a written reflection using her preferred model, which is currently that of Gibbs (1988). Sally realises that she is now building up a useful record of her CPD activity and that she needs to develop a portfolio in order to house and organise her records. She still has the one she developed at university and decides to retrieve this from her loft, look at how it was structured and decide if this is the way she needs to continue. While looking through this portfolio, she removes all the out-of-date information, retaining only material that is still current (such as certificates of academic qualifications and her merit award for practice education at university). Sally's CV will need updating before it is included and the rest of the information is archived. She has not yet decided how to structure her portfolio and therefore uses the current system to file her new TRAMm Tracker, TRAMm Trails and supervision logs. Sally has now updated her TRAMmCPD entry from Chapter 4 (see Figure 5.2, p. 70) on her TRAMm Tracker to reflect her achievements and plans. In the TRAMm Trail for her rotation into neurorehabilitation, Sally decides to enter her plans alongside those aspects she has already achieved, using italics to distinguish her plans from her achievements. As her plans are fulfilled and completed, she can easily update her Trail by removing the italics and changing the wording from future to past tense.

Tasks

The following tasks will encourage you to consider the most effective ways to record information, reflecting your own learning and retrieval style. A CPD portfolio format will be suggested and you will be encouraged to complete at least one reflection using a reflective model template and one record using a TRAMm Trail.

1. Choose a reflective model that you are less confident about using and complete one reflection for your most recent significant piece of CPD.

2. If you have not already done so, download a TRAMm Tracker from www.TRAMmCPD.com and begin to complete it for your most recent pieces of CPD.

3. If you have not already done so, download a TRAMm Trail from www.TRAMmCPD.com and begin to complete it for your most significant piece of recent CPD. (Remember to record in the 'Plan of Action' section a date and time when you will update your reflection.)

4. If you have already initiated a TRAMm Tracker and/or TRAMm Trail, remember that they have been designed to be used as 'working' documents, to be updated regularly as your learning progresses. Are you able to add to your TRAMm Tracker and/or TRAMm Trail? Have you identified further learning needs? Will you discuss this in your next supervision? Read Chapter 9 for further information.

5. If you already have a CPD portfolio, look at how it is structured, to see if it is the most effective way to organise your material. If you are happy with it, go through each of the sections and remove/archive any information that does not relate to the last two years, with the exception of information that is always relevant, such as academic qualifications or evidence of specialist/advanced practice/courses.

6. If you do not already have a CPD portfolio, investigate the available options and begin to set one up.

7. If you do not already know, find out when your next HCPC audit dates are from https://www.hcpc-uk.org/registration/registration-renewals/when-to-renew/

8. Read Chapter 8 to learn more about how you might apply your learning in practice.

A Strategic Guide to Continuing Professional Development for Health and Care Professionals:
THE TRAMm Model

Figure 7.2 TRAMm Tracker, page 1: HCPC standards and TRAMm Stations

Standard 1	Standard 2	Standard 3	Standard 4
Maintain a **continuous**, **up to date** and **accurate** record of CPD activities	Demonstrate CPD activities are a **mixture of learning activities relevant** to current or future practice	Seek to ensure that CPD has contributed to the **quality** of their practice and service delivery	Seek to ensure that CPD **benefits** the service user

Standard 5 - Only applies when called for HCPC audit
Upon request, present a written profile of own work, supported by evidence, which explains how standards have been met

TRAMm STATIONS – Suggestions only

TELL (T)	RECORD (R)	Apply (A)	MONITOR (M)	mEASURE (m)
• Informal/Formal	• Publications	• New knowledge is used in practice	• Reflective process	• Appraisal/Individualised goals achieved
• Planning in supervision	• Service Evaluation/Benchmarking	• Utilise/teach a new skill	• Formal/Informal mentorships	• Performance indicators
• Disseminating information	• Audit	• Implement a new intervention/way of working	• Supervision staff/students	• Letters of commendation
• Facilitating training sessions	• Reflection (written/recorded)	• Change in approach/values/behaviour	• Student Educator	• Standards of proficiency achieved
• Presentations	• Learning contracts	• Use up-to-date evidence to inform practice	• Establishing development plans	• Skill acquisition and improvement
• Journal club	• TRAMm Tracker/Trail	• Design an intervention evidence chart	• Peer reviews	• Audit
• Peer supervision	• Annual appraisal paperwork	• Assess financial impact of your learning	• Annual appraisal process	• Outcome measures
• Annual Appraisals/IPR/PDR	• Portfolio/Online digital curation	• Stop doing something/do something differently as a result of new knowledge	• Performance indicators	• Research/quality improvement
• Verbal reflection	• Information leaflets	• Introduce new policies/procedures/strategies	• Formative assessment	• Anecdotal: Increased confidence/time
	• Curriculum Vitae (CV)		• Competences	
	• Case notes			

Figure 7.3 Blank TRAMm Tracker, page 2

Col 1 Date	Column 2 Activity description	Certificate	Reflection	TRAMm Trail	Column 6 HCPC Standards					Column 7 TRAMm stations					Col 8 Index	Column 9 Notes
					1	2	3	4	5	T	R	A	M	m		

A Strategic Guide to Continuing Professional Development for Health and Care Professionals:
THE TRAMm Model

Figure 7.4 Blank TRAMm Trail

Please note: The TRAMm Trail has been designed for you to plan and record in a little more depth your most significant pieces of CPD. It is not anticipated that you will complete this for every piece of your CPD; only those you feel may be useful for evidence if called by the HCPC for audit. Please ensure that you maintain confidentiality.

TRAMm Trail Activity   Date: DD/MM/YY

TELL (T)	RECORD (R)	APPLY (A)

MONITOR (M)	mEASURE (m)	HCPC Standards met: (standards you aim to achieve) / PLAN of ACTION

112

Figure 7.5 Strategic TRAMm Trail

TRAMm Trail

Please note: The TRAMm Trail has been designed for you to plan and record in a little more depth your most significant pieces of CPD. It is not anticipated that you will complete this for every piece of your CPD; only those you feel may be useful for evidence if called by the HCPC for audit. Please ensure that you maintain confidentiality.

TRAMm Trail Title: Chapter 7: Strategic CPD Plan   **Date: DD/MM/YY**

These are only suggestions; you are not expected to include all these items and there may be other others that are more relevant to you

TELL (T)	RECORD (R)	APPLY (A)
<ul><li>Who do you need to share your plans with? Will you tell them formally or informally?</li><li>Who will you disseminate information to and how? Locally/nationally/globally?</li><li>Verbal reflection? Who with?</li><li>How will you disseminate your learning? Consider all the relevant stakeholders, including people who access your service, your team, manager, organisation and wider</li><li>Informal and/or formal mechanisms?</li><li>Other?</li></ul>(Include dates when these will be achieved by)	<ul><li>What record of evidence of your learning and development do you have?</li><li>Written reflection? Which model and method of reflection?</li><li>Presentation/Leaflet</li><li>Case notes</li><li>CPD portfolio updated?</li><li>Curriculum Vitae updated?</li><li>Job application completed?</li><li>Social media record</li><li>TRAMm Tracker initiated/updated?</li><li>TRAMm Trail initiated/updated?</li><li>Business plan written?</li><li>Learning contract?</li><li>Journal reading record</li><li>Critical appraisal tool</li><li>Intervention evidence chart</li><li>SWOT analysis</li><li>Mind map</li><li>Other?</li></ul>(Include dates when these will be achieved by)	<ul><li>Is it appropriate to apply your learning now or do you need to find more information?</li><li>What are you going to do next to apply what you have learnt?</li><li>Do you need permission before you implement anything new in practice? Who do you need to contact? How are you going to find their contact details?</li><li>What do you need to set up or put in place?</li><li>What information is already available to you? Where is it? How will you access it?</li><li>Can you identify further training events/journal articles/conferences/social media opportunities to support the application of your learning?</li><li>Can you teach someone else new skills that demonstrate your understanding and application in practice?</li><li>Other?</li></ul>(Include dates when these will be/are achieved by)

continued overleaf

A Strategic Guide to Continuing Professional Development for Health and Care Professionals:
THE TRAMm Model

continued from previous page

MONITOR (M)	mEASURE (m)	HCPC Standards met: *(standards you aim to achieve)*
<ul><li>Do you already monitor your progress? If so, how? If not...</li><li>How will you monitor your progress? Are there resources that could assist you?</li><li>Did you identify new learning that you achieved as your experience progressed or did this lead you to identify areas where you need to develop in the future?</li><li>Will you be supervised or mentored by anyone, formally or informally? If so, who? If not, why not? Is this a point to consider for your future Plan of Action?</li><li>If you were supervised/mentored, did you find this useful? Were you able to identify points for your future development?</li><li>Are there any monitoring roles you already undertake or could undertake (e.g. as a Mentor or Placement Educator)?</li><li>What are your strengths/learning needs in this area? What opportunities are available to help you develop your role?</li><li>Other?</li></ul>(Include dates when these will be achieved by)	<ul><li>What are you going to measure?</li><li>How will you measure your progress?</li><li>What is your baseline?</li><li>Have you achieved what you set out to achieve or has something changed? Has the outcome been different from what you anticipated? Positive or negative? Have you reflected on this?</li><li>What would you do differently next time?</li><li>Will this learning contribute to the quality of your practice/service delivery (HCPC Standard 3)?</li><li>Will this learning benefit your service user/s (HCPC Standard 4)?</li><li>Other?</li></ul>(Include dates when these will be achieved	**PLAN of ACTION**<ul><li>As you work through the TRAMm stations, what points have you identified that need to be carried out next?</li><li>What would you like to achieve next?</li><li>Where may/will this learning event lead?</li><li>Have you identified any other relevant training events journal articles/conferences/social media opportunities?</li><li>How will you ensure that you are carrying out a mixture of learning activities?</li><li>What do you need to set up or put in place?</li><li>What information is already available to you?</li><li>Update your TRAMm Tracker (timescale)</li><li>Update your TRAMm Trail (timescale)</li><li>Review and update Reflection (timescale)</li><li>What are you going to do next?</li><li>Other?</li></ul>(Include dates when these will be achieved by)

Figure 7.6 Sally's updated TRAMm Tracker

Date	Activity description	Certificate	Reflection	TRAMm Trail	HCPC Standards 1	2	3	4	5	T	R	A	M	m	Index	Notes
DD/MM/YY	Self-directed learning – planning for rotation into neurorehabilitation		R	T	1	2				T	R					See TRAMm Trail: Rotation into neurological rehabilitation. Stored on CPD memory stick
DD/MM/YY	Preceptorship completed		R		1	2	3	4		T	R	A	M	m		All documentation stored in Preceptorship file
DD/MM/YY	Introduced to TRAMmCPD by a colleague in a staff meeting			T	1	2	3	4		T	R	A	M	m	3	Learning about TRAMmCPD, organised and presented information to team colleagues. Details in TRAMm Trail
DD/MM/YY	National Professional Conference Day 2	C			1	2					R				2	Attended Stroke Rehabilitation Seminar. Conference attendance certificate in CPD file
DD/MM/YY	Attended National Professional Conference Day 1	C			1	2					R				1	Viewed poster display and exhibition; attended Professional use of Social Media session – useful information stored in CPD file

A Strategic Guide to Continuing Professional Development for Health and Care Professionals:
THE TRAMm Model

TRAMm Trail

Please note: The TRAMm Trail has been designed for you to plan and record in a little more depth your most significant pieces of CPD. It is not anticipated that you will complete this for every piece of your CPD; only those you feel may be useful for evidence if called by the HCPC for audit. Please ensure that you maintain confidentiality.

Figure 7.7 Sally's TRAMm Trail Planning for rotation into neurorehabilitation
The entries in italics are what Sally is planning to do

TRAMm Trail Title: Chapter 7: Planning for rotation into neurorehabilitation   Date: DD/MM/YY

TELL (T)	RECORD (R)	APPLY (A)
• *Discuss preparation plans for rotation into neurorehabilitation with existing Supervisor. Plan of action agreed DD/MM/YY* • *Discuss with colleagues on Stroke Unit, requesting any useful reading, assessments used and information about the most up-to-date techniques by DD/MM/YY* • *Discuss with Band 5 who is completing her 6-month rotation in neurorehabilitation by DD/MM/YY*	• *Supervision record (DD/MM/YY)* • *TRAMm Tracker updated (ongoing)* • *Initiate TRAMm Trail by DD/MM/YY* • *Notes will be taken from NICE guidelines, Care Pathway and COT Guidance, noting any questions to ask once rotation has commenced stored on USB stick by DD/MM/YY* • *Write Reflection (using Gibbs Cycle of Reflection) about forthcoming rotation by DD/MM/YY and update in six months' time*	• *New knowledge will be used to inform my practice, details to be included as I progress*

MONITOR (M)	mEASURE (m)	HCPC Standards met: 1, 2
• *Review aims and objectives set at next Supervision (DD/MM/YY)* • *Review Strategic Plan Trail at next Supervision (DD/MM/YY)*	• *Future supervision records will identify increased confidence, knowledge and skills* • *Positive feedback from service users and supervisor*	**PLAN of ACTION**

How do you record your CPD plans and activities? TRAMm Station R: RECORD

TRAMm Trail

Please note: The TRAMm Trail has been designed for you to plan and record in a little more depth your most significant pieces of CPD. It is not anticipated that you will complete this for every piece of your CPD; only those you feel may be useful for evidence if called by the HCPC for audit. Please ensure that you maintain confidentiality.

Figure 7.8 Sally's TRAMm Trail: TRAMmCPD

TRAMm Trail Title: Chapter 7: TRAMmCPD　　　　　　　　　　　　**Date: DD/MM/YY**

TELL (T)	RECORD (R)	APPLY (A)
• Informal discussion with colleagues about CPD and HCPC requirements (DD/MM/YY – ongoing) • Presented TRAMmCPD to AHP colleagues and CPD support group set up (DD/MM/YY) • Formal discussion with Manager in Supervision (DD/MM/YY)	• Emailed TRAMmCPD, requested copy of presentation and to be added to their contact list (DD/MM/YY) • Copy of TRAMmCPD Presentation and Trackers and Trails in CPD file (Index no.) • TRAMm Tracker initiated (DD/MM/YY) • TRAMm Trail updated (DD/MM/YY) • Supervision record (DD/MM/YY) • Written reflection using Gibbs Model of Reflection (DD/MM/YY)	• Applied learning through organising and presenting to colleagues (DD/MM/YY) • Teaching colleagues about TRAMmCPD and HCPC requirements (ongoing) • Organising CPD portfolio to reflect engagement in CPD (ongoing) • CPD peer support group set up (DD/MM/YY) • New entry in TRAMm Tracker for rotation into neurorehabilitation (DD/MM/YY) and TRAMm Trail initiated (DD/MM/YY) and regularly updated for rotation into neurorehabilitation (ongoing)

MONITOR (M)	mEASURE (m)	*HCPC Standards met: 1, 2 ,3, 4* **PLAN of ACTION** • *Update Reflection in 6 months* • *Update TRAMm Tracker weekly* • *Update/initiate TRAMm Trail for significant CPD*
• Formal discussion with Manager in Supervision (DD/MM/YY) • Self-monitoring and review of progress (ongoing) • TRAMm Tracker updated (DD/MM/YY)	• Positive feedback from colleagues re presentation (DD/MM/YY)	

117

8

How can you apply your learning? TRAMm Station A: Apply

Using professional/clinical reasoning to apply learning in practice is a key element within CPD; and it is important to consider the application of new knowledge and learning in relation to a variety of stakeholders. The many ways in which you may use your professional reasoning to apply your learning in practice are explored in this chapter.

The importance of applying learning in practice has always been implicit within the TRAMm Model (Hearle, Lawson & Morris 2016). Following the results of our research (Hearle & Lawson 2019, Lawson & Hearle 2019a, 2019b, Lawson 2018), it became clear that using new knowledge and skills in practice is a key element of CPD that requires more explicit reference within the TRAMm Model. To reflect this importance TRAMmCPD has been updated – Station A is now 'APPLY'.

Tasks at the end of the chapter will encourage you to consider the ways in which your learning can be applied/implemented in practice and highlight important considerations when doing this. You will also be encouraged to identify ways to analyse and explain the impact of the application.

What do we mean by 'Application' and why is it important?

Health and care regulatory bodies stipulate the need to evidence application as part of their audit process (HCPC 2019b, NMC 2019). Broughton and Harris (2019) also highlight the importance of applying your learning in practice to benefit not only yourself but also your service users, your team, organisation and wider stakeholders. Within TRAMmCPD, 'Apply' means that your new learning, knowledge and skills are used, implemented and integrated into your practice, bridging the gap between theory, research and practice. Your practice is changed or developed in some way through knowledge translation and integration into your work (Hearle & Lawson 2019, Lawson & Hearle 2019a, 2019b, Lawson 2018).

Various terms are used which help to explain what is meant by application. These include implementation (Halle, Mylopoulos, et al. 2018), knowledge translation (Barry, Kuijer-Siebelink, et al. 2017, Halle, Mylopoulos, et al. 2018, Myers, Schaefer, et al. 2017), practice change (Berndt, Murray, et al. 2017) and integration into practice (Brangan, Quinn, et al. 2015). Whichever term is used, the focus is on learning being used and applied in practice.

It is important to engage in CPD to ensure that you are up to date with current knowledge, skills and evidence (Hearle & Lawson 2019). If you then fail to apply your learning in practice, the time and effort spent is often wasted, and opportunities to develop practice may be missed. This goes against all professional codes of practice. Central to CPD is the application of new knowledge and learning in relation to yourself, the people who access your service, your team, organisation and others, in order to improve and/or change practice (Broughton & Harris 2019, Lawson 2018).

Maintaining and/or improving practice quality to benefit service users is usually the overarching aim of undertaking CPD (HCPC 2017a). However, CPD activity often fails to translate into better practice and it is widely accepted that many health and care professionals do not make sufficient use of evidence. This reluctance leads to inefficiency and ineffectiveness in delivering services (Davis, Evans, et al. 2003, Straus, Tetroe, et al. 2009, Legare, Borduas, et al. 2011). Despite this, government policy makers and many professional health and care bodies appear to be in little doubt that undertaking CPD leads to an improvement in patient outcomes. It is therefore useful to consider ways in which our learning from CPD can actually be applied to benefit ourselves, as well as the people who access our services and organisations.

Perceived barriers to application of learning

Our research suggests that there are many perceived barriers in practice which can make it challenging to apply and implement learning. The context in which you practise, and the workplace culture, can help or hinder the application of your new knowledge. Your professional reasoning, decisions, practice and changes you consider making may be based on experience and conventions and traditions within your team and workplace, rather than new knowledge from CPD, research based on evidence (Halle, Mylopoulos, et al. 2018, Welch & Dawson 2006) or informed by evidence (Taylor 2014). A lack of resources, negative workplace culture and unsupportive management may all contribute to reluctance to apply learning in practice (Penman 2014, Lowe, Rappolt, et al. 2007).

Planning, sharing and learning with others (both face-to-face and virtual) can help you to become more aware of when learning is happening (see Chapters 2, 3 and 6). Active discussions, listening and collaborating with others, in a supportive environment, can then help you to translate your learning into practice. A supportive atmosphere and opportunities to try out your new skills and knowledge with colleagues within your workplace can help you apply learning in practice.

People often refer to lack of time and resources as reasons for not engaging in CPD. In the past, one half-day per month was suggested (RCN 2007) as a reasonable amount of time for employers to allow employees for working towards their CPD. Recent guidelines (Broughton & Harris 2019) are not as specific; they place the responsibility for CPD and lifelong learning with you, whilst acknowledging that your employer has a responsibility to provide you with support in addition to statutory and mandatory training requirements. This makes it even more important to recognise and exploit all opportunities for learning that are available to you, to avoid excessive use of your own time.

How do you know if you are applying new knowledge and skills appropriately?

Once you have found a way to overcome any barriers, it is vital to ensure that you apply your learning correctly and appropriately. You may come away feeling enthusiastic and motivated (see 'the bull in a china shop' in Chapter 5), wanting to try out a new skill that you have learnt or read about. However, your learning may not have provided you with all the knowledge and skills required, or you may have misinterpreted what you have heard or read. For instance, the use of social media for CPD has increased (Bodell, Hook, et al. 2009, Hughes 2018, Murray & Ward 2017, Rushton, Gorry, et al. 2016). This provides access to many new learning opportunities but the information provided may be unsubstantiated and of poor quality in terms of its evidence base. Some professionals may lack the confidence and skills needed to assess the credibility of information, and critically evaluate and utilise research and evidence in practice (Brangan, Quinn & Spirtos 2015, Welch & Dawson 2006).

Before applying any new knowledge or skills in practice, use your professional reasoning skills and consider the following points:

- Is what you have learnt from a credible source? For example, is it from a peer-reviewed journal or professional body or have you heard about it from a friend; see Turner (2014), a website that offers a useful guide to assessing the credibility of information
- What does the evidence say? Carry out background research and reading into the subject area (see Evidence Intervention Chart, Table 8.1, p. 124)
- Reflect on the appropriateness/relevance of the information for your practice
- Practice new skills whilst new learning is fresh in your mind
- If risk is an issue (e.g. learning new moving and handling skills) it may be useful to practice on your peers or in simulated settings before testing your new skills on actual service users
- Discuss your understanding of your learning with others
- In some instances, you may need permission from others before applying your learning
- You may need further specialist training before you can apply your new knowledge, e.g. Dialectical Behaviour Therapy, non-medical prescribing, capacity assessment
- Ensure that you use the correct language/terms – for example, attending a workshop on cognitive behavioural therapy does not make you a cognitive behavioural therapist
- Initially it may be helpful to work alongside someone considered to be an expert, before applying new skills on your own
- Consider sustainability – will your service user be able to sustain the intervention when you are no longer involved? Will other staff be able to continue your project? Will funding continue?

You should only proceed once you are sure it is appropriate to use your new knowledge and skills in practice.

How to 'Apply' your learning in practice

When you have confirmed that you have the appropriate knowledge and skills, there are a variety of ways you may apply your learning in practice, depending on the area in which you work. It is also important to learn from mistakes or things that have not gone as well as you expected (Johnson Coffelt & Gabriel 2017, HCPC 2017a). Methods of applying your learning include:

- Using new knowledge/evidence to inform your practice, e.g. you stop doing something and/or do something differently as a result of new knowledge
- Utilising and/or teaching others a new skill
- Implementing a new intervention/way of working
- Changing your approach/values/behaviour
- Assessing the impact of your learning
- Introducing new policies/procedures/strategy
- Contributing to wider organisation/professional body standards, frameworks and guidance.

Application in practice can be subtle, less tangible and not always easy to notice. You may apply your learning intuitively rather than through a conscious, considered process. Recognising that learning has happened, and how it affects or impacts your practice, can be difficult (Barry, Kuijer-Siebelink, et al. 2017, Johnson Coffelt & Gabriel 2017; Berndt, Murray, et al. 2017, Brangan, Quinn & Spirtos 2015, Haywood, Pain, et al. 2013, Gibbs 2011) but it is an important skill to develop (Lawson 2018).

Several authors have attempted to provide guidance on how to recognise the impact of CPD and lifelong learning. Delors (1996, p. 92) identified four pillars of lifelong learning and education, highlighting aspects that people need to consider when undertaking CPD (rather than simply focusing on the acquisition of new knowledge). These four pillars may help to guide you in how to apply your learning in practice but it is important to note that they are different from the four Pillars of Practice identified in earlier chapters in this book:

1. 'Learning to know' means mastering learning tools. You could ask yourself, for example, 'How have I developed in the way that I have, and what has helped me?' or 'What learning tools do I have at my disposal?'

2. 'Learning to do' means gaining the skills needed for the current and future workplace. Here you could ask yourself 'What new skills have I learnt and how will they help me improve the care of my patients/service users? Where is my evidence for this?'

3. 'Learning to live together and with others' involves, for example, conflict resolution and respecting the influence of other cultures. In this case, you might ask yourself 'What knowledge and skills have I developed that will help me to work with or manage others, or work in complex situations? How can I demonstrate that I have put these into practice?'

4. 'Learning to be' means learning that contributes to your complete development. This might include your professional or other higher education qualifications, which address more than just knowledge and skills. In these circumstances, growth is often both personal and professional so you may ask yourself, 'How have I changed the way I practise as a professional? What elements of my practice demonstrate my growth in confidence?'

Another concept that appears to assist this understanding is 'knowledge translation'. This is a Canadian term that describes bridging the gap between theory and practice (Straus, Tetroe, et al. 2009). According to the Canadian Institutes of Health Research (CIHR 2005), knowledge translation involves all the CPD steps, from the creation of new knowledge to its application to ensure benefits for society, and is defined by CIHR (2005, p. 1) as

> a dynamic and iterative process that includes the synthesis, dissemination, exchange and ethically sound application of knowledge to improve health, promote more effective health services and products and a strengthened health care system.

Authors writing on this subject consider that knowledge translation provides a holistic framework in healthcare, encompassing both continuing education and CPD, and focusing on using high-quality evidence to change health outcomes (Davis, Evans, et al. 2003, Legare, Borduas, et al. 2011).

Knowledge translation has many definitions but usually includes the following criteria:

1. It occurs in the practice or clinical setting, rather than a classroom or other simulated learning environment

2. It has an explicit (and justified) need for change in health outcome or behaviour, involving the agreement of all potential stakeholders

3. It involves a process of knowledge creation, inquiry, synthesis and creation of tools, reflecting the needs of all potential stakeholders, including service users and carers

4. It includes a toolkit, guideline, checklist or pathway that has synthesised and translated recent, high-quality and reliable evidence into unambiguous techniques for practical application

5. It has a clear process for evaluating knowledge application and for ensuring continued activity.

Cusick and McCluskey (2000) stress the importance of applying evidence-based practice to improve clinical effectiveness. In order to do this, they recommend a range of strategies, including:

- Changing practitioners' or stakeholders' (such as service users' or managers') behaviour and/or expectations
- Using theory to inform the effective integration of learning into practice (such as knowledge translation)
- Developing organisational requirements for the application of evidence-based practice
- Supporting professional association initiatives and the development of clinical guidelines.

Following these criteria and strategies should enable you to plan and use your learning appropriately towards your CPD.

To assist you in translating your knowledge into practice, try putting together an intervention evidence chart for a CPD activity. This type of chart lists the evidence for the way you are using the intervention or activity and it could look something like Table 8.1.

Table 8.1 Sample intervention evidence chart

Intervention	Application	Evidence (*fictitious*)
Mindfulness	X sessions in total X mins per session Practice x times per week Depression/Anxiety X age group	Smith, A. and Jones, B. (2015). Undertaking mindfulness with people with depression and/or anxiety: A systematic Review. *Journal of XXXXXX.* 1(4), 238–56.
	X technique Closed group Maximum 6 people Depression	Green, Z. (2014). Using XXXXXX technique to enable mindfulness for people with depression. *Journal of XXXXXX.* 13(3), 134–45

The tasks at the end of this chapter encourage you to consider how to develop this idea further.

How do you demonstrate that you have 'applied' your learning?

It can sometimes be difficult to provide evidence that you have been applying your learning. However, if you have been supported by others (either financially and/or time provided), and the activity has been linked to objectives in your Professional Development Review (PDR)/Appraisal or audit/revalidation, you will be required to evidence this in some way.

These are some suggestions as to how you may be able to evidence the application of your learning in practice and you will find further ideas in other chapters in this book:

1. Your manager or peers notice a change in your practice which can be directly attributed to your learning/professional development
2. Learning leads to a successful outcome – for example, a peer-reviewed presentation, patient outcomes show improvement, you feel more confident in an area of practice
3. You can demonstrate and articulate how your practice is informed by evidence
4. Service users are offered a new assessment/intervention
5. A new way of working has been introduced as a result of your CPD
6. You complete a TRAMm Trail which shows where your learning has been applied

7. You demonstrate or teach someone else what you have learnt

8. You discover your learning has raised more questions to which you need answers prior to progressing further

9. You produce a written reflection or case study showing how your thinking or practice has changed or developed

10. Supervision records can highlight how you have applied your learning in practice.

For information on additional ways of evidencing application of your learning, please see Chapters 9 (Monitor) and 10 (measure).

Case study: Sally applies her learning in practice

In Chapter 1 we introduced Sally (an occupational therapist) who attended a two-day conference. Sally has considered the types of activities she is undertaking (Chapter 2), how to change her CPD mindset (Chapter 3) and identified her strengths and preferred learning style (Chapter 4). She then familiarised herself with TRAMmCPD (Chapter 5) and began planning, disseminating (Chapter 6) and recording her learning (Chapter 7). Sally has now rotated into neurorehabilitation, which she is enjoying.

Sally checks her social media account and sees that her professional body has posted information about new guidance they have launched about neurorehabilitation and the management of long-term conditions. She bookmarks the guidance to read in full later in the day. She downloads, reads and makes notes about how the information could be implemented within her workplace; and she plans to discuss this in her next supervision. She prints the guidance and highlights the relevant sections for her supervisor. Her supervisor agrees that some aspects could be implemented within the team. She suggests that Sally integrates current NICE guidelines, professional guidelines and National Care Pathway information to present at the next team-learning lunch. This will be a good opportunity to disseminate the information and design guidelines as to how it can be applied to guide the team's practice.

One of Sally's goals was to develop a greater understanding of how to apply neurodevelopmental approaches. Sally is now beginning to feel more confident about working with her service users in neurorehabilitation; and she has been able to explain to a new student about some of the intervention approaches to practice and how she is using them. The student has asked Sally to explain in more detail how she applies each individual approach. Sally attempts to explain but realises that the student is not clearly understanding the differences and overlaps between the approaches. This challenges Sally's thinking; she needs to be able to provide useful and easy-to-use information for this student (and future students) to assist and encourage their learning. In discussion with her supervisor, Sally agrees to collate a learning resource to support future students and new staff.

Sally updates her TRAMm Tracker and TRAMm Trail to reflect how she applied her learning from her social media use. Sally also updates her neurorehabilitation TRAMm Trail.

Tasks

These questions encourage you to think about the important considerations that enable you to apply your learning effectively and efficiently as an important element of your CPD engagement. After reflecting on these, you can read on to find out more about how to 'Monitor' and 'measure' your progress and how TRAMmCPD can help you with your CPD.

1. How do you know that you have learnt something which may be useful in your practice? Record this on your TRAMm Trail.

2. Reflect on your most recent learning activity. Have you done your background research to ensure you have the correct understanding of what you are about to apply?

3. Can you highlight one CPD activity where you have applied your learning? If so, how? If not, what could you do to ensure that this learning becomes CPD?

4. Design an intervention evidence chart (see Table 8.1) to provide a framework for one intervention/treatment/session.

5. For more information about how to encourage knowledge translation within your department/organisation, read the following article to get you started: Legare, F., Borduas, F., MacLeod, A., Sketeris, I., Campbell, B. & Jacques, A. (2011). Partnerships for knowledge translation and exchange in the context of continuing professional development. *Journal of Continuing Education in the Health Professions.* **33**(3), 181–87. doi: 10.1002/chp.20125

6. Consider the various ways in which you apply your learning in your practice: could these be expanded?

7. How can you share (Station T 'Tell') your application of your new knowledge with others within your team/learning community? Plan to do this on at least one occasion.

8. Update your TRAMm Tracker.

9. Update the 'Apply' section of your TRAMm Trail in relation to one aspect of your CPD.

10. Read Chapter 9 to find out more about how to 'Monitor' your progress.

Figure 8.1 Sally's updated TRAMm Tracker
Entries in blue are updates from previous chapter.

Date	Activity description	Certificate	Reflection	TRAMm Trail	HCPC Standards 1	2	3	4	5	TRAMm T	R	A	M	m	Index	Notes
DD/MM/YY	Self-directed learning – Rotation into neurorehabilitation		R	T	1	2	3	4		T	R	A	M	m		Details in TRAMm Trail: Neurorehabilitation. Stored on CPD memory stick.
DD/MM/YY	Preceptorship		R		1	2	3	4		T	R	A	M	m		All documentation stored in Preceptorship file
DD/MM/YY	Introduced to TRAMmCPD by a colleague in a staff meeting			T	1	2	3	4		T	R	A	M	m	3	Learning about TRAMmCPD, organised and presented information to team colleagues. Details in TRAMmCPD TRAMm Trail
DD/MM/YY	National Professional Conference Day 2	C			1	2					R	A			2	Attended Stroke Rehabilitation Seminar. Conference attendance certificate in CPD file. Information from Stroke seminar included in TRAMm Trail Neurorehabilitation
DD/MM/YY	Attended National Professional Conference Day 1	C			1	2					R				1	Viewed poster display and exhibition; attended Professional use of Social Media session – useful information stored in CPD file

A Strategic Guide to Continuing Professional Development for Health and Care Professionals:
THE TRAMm Model

TRAMm Trail

Please note: The TRAMm Trail has been designed for you to plan and record in a little more depth your most significant pieces of CPD. It is not anticipated that you will complete this for every piece of your CPD; only those you feel may be useful for evidence if called by the HCPC for audit. Please ensure that you maintain confidentiality.

TRAMm Trail Title: Chapter 8 Neurorehabilitation   Date: DD/MM/YY

TELL (T)	RECORD (R)	APPLY (A)
• Discussed preparation plans for rotation into neurorehabilitation with existing Supervisor. Plan of action agreed DD/MM/YY • Informal discussion with colleagues on Stroke Unit requesting any useful reading or information about neurodevelopmental approaches (DD/MM/YY/ – ongoing) • Practice guidelines presented to team (DD/MM/YY)	• Notes written on core principles and differences between neurodevelopmental approaches to intervention (DD/MM/YY) • Notes of questions to ask regarding NICE guidelines, Care Pathway and Professional Guidance stored on USB (DD/MM/YY) • Supervision record documenting discussions (DD/MM/YY) • Case notes (ongoing) • Written Reflection using Gibbs Model of Reflection (DD/MM/YY) • TRAMm Tracker and Trail updated (ongoing)	• Taught a student about neurodevelopmental approaches and demonstrated how they are applied in practice (DD/MM/YY) • Improved knowledge used to increase skills when using specific neuro-developmental approaches with service users (ongoing) See individual service user case notes for details.

MONITOR (M)	mEASURE (m)	HCPC Standards met: 1, 2, 3, 4 **PLAN of ACTION**
• Formal discussion of learning in Supervision with manager, reviewed TRAMm Tracker, TRAMm Trail and aims and objectives (DD/MM/YY) • Reflection in action (Sally realises how much her confidence is growing)	• Written feedback (supervision record) received from manager, highlighting good understanding of approaches and application in practice (DD/MM/YY) • Anecdotal evidence – positive verbal feedback received from service users (DD/MM/YY) • Increasing confidence in the use and understanding of neurodevelopmental approaches • Service users' results from Standardised outcome measures (DD/MM/YY)	• *Information from NICE guidelines, Care Pathway and Professional Guidance integrated into new updated Practice guidelines (DD/MM/YY)* • *Design a learning resource for new staff and students (DD/MM/YY)* • *Update TRAMm Tracker and TRAMm Trail (ongoing)* • *Update Reflection after 6 months*

Figure 8.2 Sally's updated TRAMm Trail rotation into neurorehabilitation

9

How do you keep track of your CPD? TRAMm Station M: MONITOR

Managers need to take a proactive role in the **CPD** of all their staff and enable agreed activities to be undertaken with clearly defined outcomes and monitoring arrangements. It is also important that individuals take some responsibility for monitoring their own **CPD**. There are several ways of monitoring CPD, such as supervision, mentorship, appraisal processes, peer review and reflection.

This chapter discusses the mechanisms for monitoring **CPD**. It explores in depth the meaning of the terms 'supervision' and 'mentorship' and considers how being a mentor, or being mentored, can support CPD. It also explores ways in which supervision and other strategies (such as peer review) may be used to keep track of personal and professional development. The final part of this chapter will explore the use of the **TRAMm Tracker and Trail** as part of the monitoring process and this will be illustrated in the case study.

Tasks at the end of the chapter will encourage you to consider the value of mentorship, supervision and appraisal processes to maximise their potential as part of your own professional development.

What do we mean by 'Monitor'?

Reviewing the growth of knowledge, skills and attitudes is an important part of personal and professional development. The annual appraisal or performance review is often cited as the only time when an individual's personal and professional development is officially reviewed. Yet, if used properly, appraisal should also be a method of reviewing progress, identifying and setting new goals, and measuring outcomes formally (see Chapter 10). While formal measurement is important, it does not remove the need for regular and timely feedback on your performance, which enables you to grow steadily, or the need for informal support from someone who can help you explore your aspirations or concerns.

In the TRAMm Model, 'Monitor' refers to this action of 'keeping track' or reviewing your progress so you can alter your approach or change direction if you find what you are doing is not meeting your learning needs. If you are in a management position, it refers to the actions you take to monitor the CPD being undertaken in your team. It can involve a range of formal and informal mechanisms (such as supervision, mentorship and peer review) and is part of a 'formative' process that helps to facilitate your CPD. In this TRAMm station M (Monitor), the term 'formative' is key: whichever monitoring mechanism is adopted, it should simply provide feedback, and not be used to provide a summative measure of performance to which some kind of reward is attached (such as promotion, salary increase or qualification). Some mechanisms can be used to monitor and measure progress; and where this is the case, the distinction will be clarified.

Why is it important to monitor progress?

Monitoring and tailoring of progress enables you to identify personal and professional strengths and needs. It is also a process whereby managers can maintain an overview of their most important and expensive resource (staff) by keeping track of the strengths and development needs of their team and organisation. There are many occasions when an individual's personal and professional development needs may be different from those of the organisation; and it is essential to be clear about these expectations to ensure that we are monitoring development appropriately.

The value of monitoring CPD for the individual

When considering the importance of monitoring, a good analogy is the education process, which we all experience during our careers. Think back to when you were at school. You will have had classes (teaching) during your studies, and exams at the end of each term or year (summative assessments), but what formative tasks and assessments did you have to support your learning? Homework, presentations and class tests were not only included for the teachers' benefit. They were also put in place to monitor your progress in understanding and ability. Doing poorly in homework or a class test did not mean that you failed the year and could not progress. It just meant that your teacher, your parents and you yourself knew where you were struggling and where further support or tuition was required to enable you to pass your exams. If you had only received classroom teaching without any monitoring, you could have wasted a whole year – and perhaps ended up failing because of problems that could have been easily addressed but were not picked up earlier, through your formative work.

As a health and care professional, the same applies during your practice or clinical placements; and if you are a health or care student, this may be something you are already familiar with. You will have had some instruction from your placement or clinical educators but, without regular and timely monitoring and feedback, you could continue to perform badly until you discovered you had failed at the end of the placement period. This would be a waste of time, not only for you but also for your placement educators. More importantly, it could cause harm or distress to patients or service users and a significant waste of money for the service. Fortunately, it is common to get regular informal feedback, observed assessments and encouragement to reflect through more formal supervision to help you recognise your strengths and make plans to address your learning needs.

If you have had a less favourable experience of placement, the main reason for this may well have been poor monitoring or feedback. If you are a student and have just had a placement, or are currently on placement, it may be useful to reflect upon your experiences of monitoring and feedback. It is also important to note that monitoring and feedback are not only undertaken to identify and rectify problems. Monitoring can also be useful to highlight and further develop a person's strengths, as can be seen in the example below.

Example 7.1 Adam, the operating department practitioner

Adam is an operating department practitioner who is six months into his first post in an orthopaedic surgical team. Adam has had to learn several new skills since commencing this role. These have been highlighted as part of his preceptorship programme and he is now beginning to recognise an increase in his confidence. His supervisor has helped him to understand the department processes, which he can now follow without supervision, and his communication skills in Recovery have been noted as excellent by the ward manager.

Recently Adam's manager has observed that Adam is particularly proactive in helping to support students whenever they are in the department. They in turn seem to respond well to his teaching and he is able to explain things clearly and concisely. This strength is discussed at Adam's next supervision. When Adam admits that teaching is something he would like to do, it is agreed that he will undertake the post-registration course on supervision of students.

Monitoring is also used to check on progress in terms of career direction. When we are undertaking our professional studies or when we are newly qualified, very few of us know exactly which area we wish to specialise in. Instead we explore a few specialist areas via rotations or several job applications until we find an area that motivates us, as a result of a clinical interest or because we find we are good at it. Even then, we may not stay in that area – either because we specialise further or we choose to change direction. (For example, perhaps moving into management or education or promotion leads us down a different path or we retrain in a different profession.)

If we review Adam in five years' time, it is possible that he will have re-evaluated his career direction and either moved to a different specialty or retrained as a theatre nurse to gain greater autonomy in surgical care. In this way, the process of monitoring and feedback helps us pursue our career aspirations and consider opportunities, reviewing our own preferences in relation to the options available to us. Career, learning and development frameworks can be useful to help us identify our areas of progress, and formulate new learning needs and future goals (see Chapter 3).

The value of monitoring CPD for the organisation

The RCN (2007) recommended that healthcare professionals received at least 45 hours per year for CPD in order to maintain competence and develop their practice to adapt to the changing needs of the service users and organisations in which they worked. Although this recommendation is not included in the updated *Principles for Continuing Professional Development and Lifelong Learning* (Broughton & Harris 2019), it is still a useful guide. Likewise, O'Sullivan (2006) highlights the value of organisations that are committed to the learning and development of their staff (see Chapter 3 on learning organisations). If they are investing substantial time and money in CPD, it follows that the organisations themselves should also want to keep a check on what their money is paying for. This is another reason why it is important to measure (see Chapter 10), and disseminate (see Chapter 6), the impact of your learning and development.

In a study exploring CPD within hospital trusts, Mathers, Mitchell & Hunn (2012) found that CPD for staff often occurred in a vacuum, with no connection to the organisation's goals or the appraisal process. In cases like this, where CPD took place in isolation, Mathers *et al.* (2012) found that there was less likelihood of it being implemented or documented. If you are a manager of staff in any organisation, this is important information, as it suggests that you may be spending your budget (in terms of CPD costs or staff time) on something for which you will never see a return and this is not the way a good business is run. The TRAMm Model emphasises these requirements in its stations, where dissemination and planning (in 'Tell') and documentation (in 'Record') are considered essential for full engagement in CPD.

Those involved in the top-level overall management of the organisation will not have time to take an interest in what each individual is undertaking for their CPD. However, senior managers need to identify the strategic direction of the organisation and they should also ensure that these goals are relayed to line managers, who will in turn reflect these within staff development plans. If you are a line manager, you will probably measure performance against objectives set as part of the appraisal process. Regardless, it is important to undertake regular monitoring so that information about your team, and how they are contributing to the organisation, can be provided when required.

As a line manager in an organisation, you could be monitoring and documenting many aspects of CPD, including:

- The range and frequency of CPD activities undertaken by those you supervise
- The number of hours each staff member has taken as CPD
- The developing range of knowledge and skills of your team
- Evidence showing how and where this CPD has been disseminated
- Information about the impact of CPD on service user outcomes
- The running costs of CPD activities undertaken
- Income generated and money saved as a direct or indirect result of staff CPD.

This list is not exhaustive but provides some guidance, following the TRAMm Model of the important CPD aspects and how they may be reviewed. Adopting TRAMmCPD for all the staff you manage could help to provide a standardised record, from which data required for the above monitoring could be easily retrieved.

How do we monitor our progress and what do we need?

There are many ways to monitor progress and encourage personal and professional development. This will also provide information for organisational monitoring, as indicated previously. The following section provides an overview of some of the most common enablers of monitoring, including:

- Supervision and clinical supervision
- Preceptorship (or equivalent)
- Mentoring
- Revisiting objectives from your appraisal
- Peer review and work-based learning as monitoring
- Self-monitoring via reflection.

Supervision and clinical supervision

Supervision is designed to provide individual staff with accountability (facilitating safe and effective practice), support and learning (O'Neill 2004). It is a requirement of practice (Gopee 2015) and in most working environments some time is allocated to facilitate supervision, although the amount of time varies according to your employer and/or supervisor.

According to the Care Quality Commission (CQC 2013, p. 4) clinical supervision is:

> 'a safe and confidential environment for staff to reflect on and discuss their work and their personal and professional responses to their work. The focus is on supporting staff in their personal and professional development and in reflecting on their practice.'

In addition, the Royal College of Occupational Therapists (COT 2010, p. 2) stated that:

> 'supervision involves learning through reviewing, reflecting and discussing the experiences of the workplace, confirming and building upon the positive events and exploring options for the less easy occurrences, so developing the practitioner's understanding of their work environment and broadening their range of personal and professional resources in terms of skills and knowledge.'

Taken together, these two definitions explain what supervision can (and cannot) be expected to achieve. The CQC (2013, pp. 3–4) identifies three main types of supervision, although the terms are often used interchangeably:

1. **Managerial supervision** is carried out by a supervisor with authority and accountability for the supervisee. It provides the opportunity for staff to:
- Review their performance
- Set priorities and objectives in line with the organisation's objectives and service needs
- Identify training and development needs.

2. **Clinical supervision** provides an opportunity for staff to:
- Reflect on their practice
- Discuss individual cases in depth
- Change or modify practice and identify training and development needs.

3. **Professional supervision** (often interchangeable with clinical supervision) is sometimes used when supervision is carried out by another member of the same profession or group. This can give staff the opportunity to:
- Review professional standards
- Keep up to date with developments in their profession
- Identify professional training and development needs
- Ensure that they are working within professional codes of conduct and boundaries.

For the purposes of this chapter, the term 'supervision' is used to refer to all the above types of supervision. Youngstrom (2009) and professional bodies, such as the Royal College of Occupational Therapists (COT 2015) and the Chartered Society of Physiotherapists (CSP 2017), acknowledge that the main aim of supervision is to achieve safe, effective and high-quality service delivery. For supervision to be effective, COT (2015), CSP (2017) and Strong (2009) highlight the need for it to be conducted in a safe and supportive manner. This is especially important, as evidence suggests that employees who experience an atmosphere of fear and distrust in the workplace are more likely to make mistakes and report them less frequently (Dixon-Woods 2010). This failure to report mistakes can not only stunt individual professional growth but also stifle organisational learning; and in the clinical field, it can potentially cause harm to service users.

In a study of allied health professionals, Strong, Kavanagh, et al. (2003) discovered that supervision helped to increase job satisfaction, effectiveness and reasoning, concurrently preventing stress and burnout, two factors that have been associated with poor patient safety (Schaufeli & Bakker 2004). Strong (2009) also identified the benefits of supervision in terms of the organisation; staff develop greater understanding of the culture and practice of the organisation and a stronger sense of organisational identity. This in turn assists both recruitment and retention.

The Royal College of Occupational Therapists (COT 2015) highlights the importance of considering context and personal preference in order to decide on the most appropriate supervision style and format. Thus, for example, in the NHS where supervision is an accepted part of practice, it is likely to follow a clinical supervision style (CQC 2013) on a one-to-one basis. In a specialist unit, where there is a small expert team, they may prefer the option of group supervision, which may also be the preferred format when teams are dealing with complex cases – as in social care. Peer supervision, or long-arm supervision, may be the style of choice when a professional is working in professional isolation or in a non-traditional or role-emerging setting. Advances in the use of technology have also seen the emergence of e-supervision, whereby meetings can take place via Skype, video-conferencing or E-discussion.

Whichever supervision style is selected, the core principles remain the same and are reflected in many books, articles and professional body statements. These principles are most effectively summarised by the Chartered Society of Physiotherapy (CSP 2017, p. 1) who state that clinical supervision should:

1. Support and enhance practice for the benefit of patients and service users
2. Develop skills in reflection to narrow the gap between theory and practice (see Chapter 7)
3. Involve a supervisor and practitioner, or group of practitioners, reflecting on and critically evaluating practice
4. Be distinct from formal line management supervision and appraisal (see Chapter 10)
5. Be planned, systematic and conducted within agreed boundaries
6. Be explicit about the public and confidential elements of the process
7. Facilitate clear and unambiguous communication, conducted in an atmosphere of beneficence (keeping the welfare of the supervisee at the centre of the process)
8. Define an outcomes-based action plan that can be more broadly developed to assist the practitioner's professional development through the appraisal process (see Chapter 2)
9. Be evaluated against set standards, from the time it is initially developed and implemented.

The clinical supervision process should:

1. Involve all individuals in the service, be signed up to by staff, and supported and resourced by management
2. Be developed in partnership with managers and practitioners
3. Be supported by appropriate resources (including time, training and replacement staff)
4. Facilitate practitioner access to their chosen model of supervision, as appropriate
5. Support a local system for supervisors to further develop their skills in facilitation
6. Be developed in parallel with collating a portfolio of learning, so that the practitioner is supported to develop and demonstrate skills of reflection and evidencing learning from experience (see Chapter 7).

As a supervisee, it is important to plan for your sessions and record a summary, together with a list of actions to be undertaken following the supervision. There are various formats for recording supervision; in TRAMmCPD, the TRAMm Tracker and Trail can help to guide both you and the session itself (see Chapter 7).

Finally, if you are acting as a supervisor, it is important to allow time to undertake the supervision and keep the issues expressed by the supervisee confidential, no matter how insignificant you may think they are. You must also access appropriate training for the role. It may only be a short course but it will certainly help to clarify your role and delineate responsibilities between yourself and the supervisee.

Mentorship and the role of the mentor

Across the healthcare professions, the term 'mentoring' is used in a variety of ways. In TRAMmCPD, mentoring is considered to be a process which encourages people to manage their own learning with the support of a 'mentor'. Through the process of mentoring individuals are facilitated to develop skills and improve performance to become the practitioner they aspire to be (Parsloe & Leedham 2009).

Mentoring differs from supervision in several ways. The mentor and mentee have a different type of relationship from a supervisor and supervisee. Although the mentor is usually more senior or experienced than the mentee, the mentor tends to adopt more of a friend or 'buddy' status. The mentor is also usually from a similar field or has similar experiences to the mentee. Ideally, the mentor should be selected by the mentee, as it is important for the mentee to have a mentor they respect and trust. The role of the mentor is to advise or support, rather than to oversee performance or direct work in accordance with organisational strategy. During mentorship sessions, the focus is on the mentee and their long-term personal and professional development.

During supervision, in contrast, the focus is usually on practice and how the individual is performing in the work context, usually taking more of a short-term view. Both have a role in ensuring that the mentee understands and engages in evidence-based practice (Gopee 2015). Mentorship sessions should ideally be directed by the needs of the mentee, with the mentee setting and leading the agenda; whereas supervision is often guided by the structure adopted in the workplace and may focus more on requirements from practice. A supervisor explores performance and practice issues; a mentor's role is to develop confidence and self-belief by asking questions and challenging thoughts and perceptions. Mentoring provides an opportunity for the mentee to explore ideas in confidence, become more self-aware and scrutinise themselves, as well as considering any issues, aspirations and potential opportunities.

Records of both supervision and mentorship are of course confidential. However, meetings with a mentor should remain strictly confidential at all times, whereas communications during supervision can be used to inform professional development and help deal with performance issues should they arise. It is therefore no surprise that the mentor and mentee can discuss any issues at all (whether personal or professional), whereas supervision generally tends to focus on work-related issues. If you do not currently have a mentor, it is well worth considering finding one.

Mentors can provide invaluable support throughout your career. They can help you think through different ways of tackling difficult situations. You can also use mentoring sessions to air concerns about your own performance or relationships at work, without fear of reprisal. Because the mentoring relationship can continue over a period of time, sessions can be invaluable as a means to facilitate self-monitoring of values, attitudes and self-image; these are issues that are difficult to reflect upon without someone to challenge you in a mutually trusting relationship.

If you feel you have the required skills and experience, becoming a mentor is also an excellent professional development opportunity and could be considered as one of your CPD activities.

Preceptorship and monitoring

Agenda for Change Final Agreement (DH 2004) was a major change for all staff in the NHS. At the same time, preceptorship was introduced as a way to support newly qualified staff and facilitate CPD through their first 6–12 months. In preceptorship, successful progress through individual professional development plans, linked to the Knowledge and Skills Framework (KSF), leads to incremental advance. This is similar to ASYE (Assessed and Supported Year in Employment) for social workers (Skills for Care 2019) or probation in other organisations.

The Department of Health (DH 2010, p. 11) defines preceptorship as:

> A period of structured transition for the newly registered practitioner during which he or she will be supported by a preceptor, to develop their confidence as an autonomous professional, define skills, values and behaviours and to continue on their journey of lifelong learning.

Preceptorship is one of the more formal monitoring mechanisms, in which the final outcome may be considered a form of measurement of CPD, like appraisal (see Chapter 8). However, the process allows for self-monitoring and monitoring of professional development by a superior. The DH (2010) identifies three contributors to the preceptorship process: the preceptee, the preceptor and the employer, each of whom has a responsibility to ensure that the process runs effectively. The employer ensures compliance with the KSF and has a responsibility to allow time for the preceptee and preceptor to meet and for professional development. The preceptor has the role of facilitating the professional development of the preceptee and providing timely and documented feedback; while the preceptee must follow the programme and take responsibility for their own learning.

There is no set format for a preceptorship programme but it is expected to involve theoretical, practical and attitudinal development. Like CPD, preceptorship learning can occur through a range of activities but the DH (2010) recommends that there should be approximately 4–6 days allocated for theoretical learning and around 18 hours for more practical learning such as reflection and practice development. The exact process is usually determined by the individual organisation to ensure equity for all new staff.

There are many benefits of preceptorship for all parties (including service users) but the main advantages are that quality of care is enhanced for the service user; the employee feels valued and has job satisfaction, with increased confidence and competence in the role (Jamieson, Harris & Hall 2012); and the preceptor invests in their own professional development by developing new skills. Professional induction and development schemes are always under review and constantly evolving; and such schemes are important to support your transition into practice.

Self-monitoring via reflection

In Chapters 2 and 7 we explored the process of reflection and a range of models to assist with it. Reflection is an excellent way to facilitate self-monitoring, particularly in relation to those aspects that are more difficult to measure, such as confidence, attitudes and values (Constable 2013).

In order to use reflection in monitoring your CPD, it is useful to undertake a reflection before you start an element of CPD – for example, at the beginning of a course or at the start of a new job or rotation. One reflection on its own can help monitor a shift in your knowledge, skills or attitudes but comparing one reflection with another can explicitly evidence a change over a period of time.

Peer review and monitoring

Peer review is appraisal of work by someone with similar competence in order to drive up quality and provide credibility. Peer review sits on the dividing line between monitoring (formative assessment to monitor progress and provide feedback) and measurement (summative assessment leading to a reward, award or outcome, depending upon its context). In this chapter we will discuss the purpose of peer review in monitoring and it will then be revisited in Chapter 10 in relation to measuring CPD.

When used for monitoring purposes, peer review is usually seen in the workplace and is often referred to as peer review in a given context – for instance, peer review of teaching or peer review of practice. In peer review of teaching, a fellow colleague will be responsible for evaluating your performance in a particular teaching situation and will provide constructive feedback. This feedback is usually kept confidential between the reviewee and reviewer, but the reviewee may choose to share the feedback in supervision or appraisal to help identify future learning needs for CPD.

Using TRAMmCPD to help you with the monitoring process

TRAMmCPD tools can help you to record and monitor your progress in various areas. The TRAMm Tracker will help you to monitor how you are meeting the HCPC standards for CPD (HCPC 2017a) and will encourage dialogue around your full engagement with the CPD process via the TRAMm stations. It will highlight shortcomings or omissions in certain areas and, when used with the TRAMm model, can show you how to work on those areas (see Chapter 7 for more detail on using this in practice).

The TRAMm Trail will allow you to map in greater depth your activities and ideas for some of the more complex cases that you may wish to discuss during the supervision process, and help you keep track of your progress on visiting the TRAMm stations. It also provides a box in which to insert your plans, to keep them readily available for monitoring purposes and for further development.

If you are using the TRAMm Trail and find you are struggling to complete the 'Monitor' station, it is possible that there is no monitoring currently taking place for this particular piece of CPD. You can now identify this as a gap in your learning and consciously decide to include monitoring in future. If you decide that monitoring *has* been taking place, ask yourself the following questions:

- Before you started undertaking this aspect of CPD, had you made a plan of what you wanted to achieve? Was this documented? Or was it a thought or reflective process? It is very difficult to monitor something when you have no idea what you are monitoring.

- Were you supervised or mentored by anyone, in a formal or informal way? If not, why not? Would this be a point to consider for your future Plan of Action? It is very difficult to undertake monitoring if you have no time, person or strategy to help with this.
- If you were supervised or mentored, did you find this useful? Were you able to identify points for your future development and what exactly helped you to do so? What evidence do you have of this? This evidence can be recorded as monitoring.
- Did you monitor your own progress? Did you identify new learning that you achieved as your experience progressed? Or did this lead to identifying areas where you needed to develop in the future? If so, exactly how did you identify these areas? If it is not clear, perhaps you should make your thoughts more explicit by undertaking a reflection to provide evidence of your monitoring. For example, you may have had some difficult discussions with a patient and family and needed to think about how you were going to approach this in the most appropriate and sensitive manner. This is about being aware of, or monitoring, your own limitations or gaps in knowledge and what to do about this. It is this type of thinking that may have led to your informal supervision or it may have set the agenda for more formal supervision.

As a supervisor, you can also use the TRAMm Tracker and Trail to structure and record supervision sessions for each individual you supervise. This ensures that you ask the same of each individual, while allowing for flexibility to reflect their particular approach to CPD.

As a manager, you could use the tools to structure the CPD for all your staff, providing a consistent mechanism for gathering the data you require in order to monitor CPD across your team or department. During the pilot stage of TRAMmCPD, several departments adopted this approach to provide a framework for their team and guide their strategy for monitoring and measuring CPD.

Case study: Sally begins to engage in the monitoring of her progress

In Chapter 1 we introduced Sally (an occupational therapist) who attended a two-day conference. Sally has considered the types of activities she is undertaking (Chapter 2), and how to change her CPD mindset (Chapter 3). She has also identified her preferred learning style (Chapter 4), familiarised herself with TRAMmCPD (Chapter 5) and begun planning, disseminating (Chapter 6) and recording her learning (Chapter 7).

After rotating into a neurorehabilitation post, Sally learnt to use TRAMmCPD to record her progress and activities, using the TRAMm Tracker and TRAMm Trail, and apply her learning in practice. Sally is now five months into her new rotation and is conscious that she has one month left before she moves into her next post in rheumatology. She is not looking forward to leaving, as she is enjoying her time in neurorehabilitation. She decides that now is a good time to discuss planning for both the forthcoming rotation and her future career pathway. She is concerned about sounding as if she is complaining to her supervisor so she decides to meet a friend for coffee, to talk it over. Her friend Joe is a psychologist, who has also been acting as her mentor over the last six months.

Joe agrees that it is important for Sally to begin to plan her career development and to use her next supervision to discuss her concerns about her forthcoming rotation and how to address this. Together they explore how Sally can do this in a constructive way. Joe advises Sally to carefully consider her aspirations for the next couple of years and says he is happy to have another chat before Sally presents her thoughts in supervision. Sally uses the following week to reflect on what Joe has said. She decides to evaluate her learning and development against the criteria of the Career Development Framework for occupational therapists and undertakes a SWOT analysis to map her current situation (see Table 9.1).

Sally emails a copy of her SWOT analysis to Joe and arranges to talk further on the telephone in a few days' time. Joe and Sally decide that Sally's proposal to her supervisor will be for her to continue into her new rotation post but also discuss ways in which she can maintain her clinical interest in neurorehabilitation. At the same time, she would like to develop her management and leadership skills to place herself in a good position to apply for any neurorehabilitation Band 6 positions in the future.

Sally decides to update her Tracker with a new entry, entitled 'Career development planning'. She initiates a new TRAMm Trail, which she will update regularly over the next 12 months or until she secures a Band 6 position.

Sally has her weekly meeting with her supervisor to discuss her caseload; they have been monitoring the progress of Sally's work with a patient with complex problems. Sally is concerned that the consultant has requested an assessment of the patient's driving skills even though she feels that this is inappropriate at this stage of the patient's rehabilitation. With her supervisor, Sally agrees that the process of driving skills is a further learning need and makes a plan to address it. She plans to document her progress on a new TRAMm Trail. Although this is theoretically part of her normal working practice, she believes that it also contributes to her CPD, as she has limited understanding in this area.

They also discuss the limited use of Gibbs as a reflective model now that Sally is clearly beginning to reflect on a regular basis. Sally suggests that she should explore other models that may help her to reflect in greater depth, such as Fish and Twinn (1997) or Rodgers (2002). During this meeting, Sally decides to approach her supervisor with her proposals regarding her future career development. Her supervisor states that she is impressed with how Sally has prepared her case and highlights Sally's professional progress over the last 12 months, confirming her support of Sally's plans.

They agree that, within the next month, Sally should set some new goals that reflect her ambitions and outline a plan for how these can be met. As part of this development plan, Sally and her manager discuss the possibility that Sally can continue with the development of a driving pathway that she has just commenced for people with neurological deficits. Her current line manager agrees to confirm this with her future new line manager in rheumatology. Sally documents this plan on her supervision record and in her new TRAMm Trail (see Figures 9.1 and 9.2, pp. 143, 144).

Table 9.1 SWOT Analysis: Sally and her profile for promotion

Strengths: Internal driving forces	**Weaknesses:** Internal restraining forces
• Contrasting clinical experience to include six months in orthopaedics, mental health and neurorehabilitation • Member of local neuro special interest group • Has undertaken a recent two-day course on CBT • Some experience of supporting students • Can search databases, evaluate and apply evidence/guidelines • Well-organised and up-to-date CPD portfolio • Clear strategic career development plan	• Lacks motivation for future rheumatology rotation as this is not an area of interest and does not fit with future career plans • No formal research experience since university • Limited management experience in relation to change, staff or finance • No Masters degree or M level study to date
Opportunities: External driving forces	**Threats:** External restraining forces
• Active, local neuro special interest group offering contribution to funding for neuro-related courses • Specialist neurorehabilitation course runs annually • Department has been asked to complete a service evaluation • In-house leadership course available on an annual basis; currently recruiting for start in six months' time • New financial year starts in four weeks and funding requests are invited for CPD • Accredited placement educators' course is run at the local university, which can be undertaken as an M level module • Rheumatology department, which regularly takes students – opportunity to further develop supervision skills	• Limited promotion opportunities and high competition in the local region • Band 6 positions now requesting management experience as desirable • Band 7 posts requiring Masters level study in addition to essential management skills • High level of competition for CPD funding within the organisation

Tasks

The following tasks are designed to facilitate your thinking around the issue of monitoring and how you will apply it to yourself. They will also encourage you to think about your own role as a mentor and how CPD can enable you to undertake the role successfully:

1. Visit your own professional body website and see if they have current guidance on any of the aspects mentioned in this chapter, such as briefings on supervision, mentorship or preceptorship. Pay particular attention to your responsibilities in whichever role you are undertaking. For instance, in the role of supervisee or supervisor, what is expected of you?

2. If you are about to start your first post or about to become a preceptor for the first time, read the preceptorship framework (DH 2010), paying particular attention to your roles and responsibilities and what you should expect from others.

3. Think about how you currently monitor your own progress. Ask yourself the following: Do I monitor how I am progressing and if so how? What objectives have been agreed within my appraisal process and am I on track to meet them? Are there things/tools/people I could use to assist me?

4. Take time to write a reflection on your most recent experience of monitoring and feedback at your workplace; or, if you are a student, on your most recent placement. Place this reflection in your portfolio.

5. If you do not have an official mentor, consider those people who you believe could help you in this way. Then make contact with one of them to see if they would be prepared to act as your mentor.

6. If you already have a mentor, reflect upon whether you are using them appropriately. Are there ways in which the relationship could work more effectively to support your personal and professional development?

7. Consider what monitoring roles you could undertake, such as mentor or placement educator. What are your own strengths and learning needs in this area and what opportunities are available to help you to develop your role? Undertake a SWOT analysis entitled 'Me as a monitor' to help you to summarise all this.

8. Continue to develop your portfolio and add to your TRAMm Tracker and Trails.

9. Read Chapter 10 to discover more about measuring your CPD (TRAMm station 'measure').

Figure 9.1 Sally's updated TRAMm Tracker. Entries in blue highlight updates from previous chapter.

Please note: Conference attendance Day 1 and 2 from Figure 8.1 have been removed here, due to space restrictions; Sally would keep these as part of her TRAMm Tracker as her chronological, up-to-date list of activities.

Date	Activity description	Certificate	Reflection	TRAMm Trail	HCPC Standards 1	2	3	4	5	TRAMm T	R	A	M	Index m	Notes
DD/MM/YY	Service development – Design new return to driving pathway				1	2				T					Conversation in Supervision
DD/MM/YY	Career Development Planning – Current skills mapped to Career Development Framework		R	T	1	2				T	R	A	M	m	See TRAMm Trail: Career Development Planning and SWOT Analysis
DD/MM/YY	Self-directed learning – Rotation into neurorehabilitation		R	T	1	2	3	4		T	R	A	M	m	Details in TRAMm Trail: Neurorehabilitation. Stored on CPD memory stick.
DD/MM/YY	Preceptorship		R		1	2	3	4		T	R	A	M	m	All documentation stored in Preceptorship file
DD/MM/YY	Introduced to TRAMmCPD by a colleague in a staff meeting			T	1	2	3	4		T	R	A	M	m 3	Learning about TRAMmCPD, organised and presented information to team colleagues. Details in TRAMmCPD TRAMm Trail

A Strategic Guide to Continuing Professional Development for Health and Care Professionals:
THE TRAMm Model

TRAMm Trail

Please note: The TRAMm Trail has been designed for you to plan and record in a little more depth your most significant pieces of CPD. It is not anticipated that you will complete this for every piece of your CPD; only those you feel may be useful for evidence if called by the HCPC for audit. Please ensure that you maintain confidentiality.

Figure 9.2 Sally's TRAMm Trail: Career Development Planning

TRAMm Trail Title: Chapter 9: Career development planning   **Date: DD/MM/YY**

TELL (T)	RECORD (R)	APPLY (A)
• Informal discussions with mentor and manager regarding career progression (DD/MM/YY)	• Mapped current skills to the Career Development Framework, results summarised in a SWOT Analysis (ongoing) • Goals explicitly recorded in supervision log (DD/MM/YY) • Reflection of current progression and future career plans using Boud model of reflection (DD/MM/YY – ongoing) • TRAMm Tracker updated (DD/MM/YY) • TRAMm Trail initiated (DD/MM/YY)	• Mapped current skills to the Career Development Framework (RCOT 2017) and results summarised in a SWOT Analysis (ongoing) • Goals explicitly recorded in supervision log (DD/MM/YY) • Greater awareness of the four Pillars of Practice within the Career Development Framework (RCOT 2017) and recognising opportunities as they arise (ongoing)
MONITOR (M)	**mEASURE (m)**	**HCPC Standards met: 1, 2**
• Meetings with Mentor to discuss and plan career development (DD/MM/YY) • Discussion and goal setting in Supervision with manager (DD/MM/YY) • Reflection of current progression and future career plans using Fish and Twinn (1997) model of reflection (DD/MM/YY – ongoing)	• Mapped current skills to the Career Development Framework and results summarised in a SWOT Analysis (ongoing)	**PLAN of ACTION** • Investigate placement educator course by DD/MM/YY • Find out more about driving assessment skills by DD/MM/YY • Investigate leadership opportunities • Update TRAMm Tracker (timescale) • Update TRAMm Trail (timescale) • Update Reflection after 3 months

10

How do you measure your CPD? TRAMm Station m: mEASURE

Remember, in TRAMm the 'm' denotes 'measure', purely to distinguish it from 'M' for 'monitor'. The lower-case 'm' does not have any significance in terms of relative importance.

Setting specific, individualised goals enables you to set a baseline upon which the success of your CPD can be evidenced and measured. This chapter discusses why measurement is a critical part of CPD, and how outcomes can be used to indicate progress and future direction. It identifies and explains mechanisms for evidencing and measuring the outcomes and impact of CPD, providing illustrations through case examples and a completed TRAMm Tracker and Trail. Suggestions for how to make your objectives specific are given.

At the end of the chapter, tasks will provide opportunities for you to develop your own measurement baselines, explore ways to measure your CPD and to practise using the TRAMmCPD tools.

What do we mean by 'measure' (m)?

In Chapter 9 we explored the concept of monitoring, which was described as a formative process that relies upon constructive feedback or self-critique to facilitate professional development. While monitoring allows individuals to grow and develop, it is no longer acceptable simply to declare that professional development is taking place. Instead we need to provide evidence to demonstrate what development has occurred, how it has taken place, and what impact it has had. This evidence is achieved by measurement, which can take a variety of forms, the most common of which will be discussed in more detail below.

Friedman (2012) describes two main types of measurement for CPD: input and output measurement. Input measurement measures the CPD undertaken – such as hours spent attending courses, credits received, and certificates awarded. However, many professional bodies have now acknowledged that these input measurements do not actually demonstrate that anything has been learnt through the CPD; nor do they show that what has been learnt will be applied in practice and lead to change.

As part of the regulation process, the HCPC (2017a) CPD standards reflect the idea of output measurement. This refers to aspects such as measures of impact or, in other words, what has been achieved as a direct result of your CPD. If you revisit the HCPC CPD standards in Chapter 1, you will remember that standards 3 and 4 relate to application and impact, which could be interpreted in several ways in the environment in which you are working. These standards relate to:

- Your service users or other stakeholders (e.g. What has been the impact on a patient's independence or a student's exam results?)
- The organisation (e.g. Can you demonstrate an improvement in delivery of service? Is there a cost saving? Are patients being discharged earlier?)
- The staff of the organisation where you work (e.g. Did you implement something that improved working conditions or made something easier for staff?)
- Yourself? (e.g. Have you noticed an increase in your confidence? Have you developed a new skill that you are now applying in practice?)

Measurement is needed at both macro and micro levels, and we need to measure successes and also learn from any failures. For your CPD to be relevant or successful, it does not necessarily have to result in an improvement. Instead it may simply highlight that something is wrong or does not work, in which case stopping it or doing something differently might indirectly lead to a positive change.

When submitting your evidence to the HCPC, they do not expect you to show that all your CPD has had significant benefits for service users. However, they will expect you to have considered why it has (or has not) benefited service users and, if appropriate, what you would do differently next time (HCPC 2017a).

Why do we need to measure CPD?

In Chapter 4 we discussed the importance of setting out your learning needs and being specific about your goals, but how do you know if you have achieved what you set out to achieve? Whether it is meeting HCPC standards, organisational targets or objectives you have set for yourself, there is no point in setting goals if you do not have some way to check that they have been met.

Since the introduction of Clinical Governance and the redefining of standards by the HCPC (2017a), CPD may cost a great deal in money and resources. As a result, CPD outcome measurement is now required by a number of organisations (including professional and regulatory bodies), as well as managers across a range of sectors responsible for service delivery and the education of health and social care professionals.

Evidence also suggests (Haywood, Pain, et al. 2012 and 2013) that managers and organisations perceive little benefit in supporting individual staff CPD when they do not see tangible evidence of its benefits for the organisation and service users; it is therefore your responsibility to make this link explicit.

The HCPC (2017a), which is responsible for the audit of CPD for their registered health and care professionals, states that CPD should not only be undertaken to influence practice but also to benefit service users. The meaning of the term 'service user' depends very much on the context in which the individual undertaking the CPD is working, as shown in Table 10.1 (below).

Table 10.1 Definition of service user versus context (HCPC 2017a)

Role	Example of work context	Service users – anyone who uses or is affected by your practice (HCPC 2017a)
Practitioner/student practitioner	Hospital/social care setting/ward/department/unit/patient's home/school/care home	People who access your service, carers, family members, colleagues, managers
Manager	Hospital/social care setting/ward/department/unit/patient's home/school/care home/professional body	Staff/colleagues, people who access your service/members/journalists/librarians/press officers/senior executives
Educator	University/placement setting	Students/colleagues/practice educators/policy makers
Researcher	University/laboratory/hospital/community	Collaborators/participants/users of research

Once you have considered your work context, it is important to think about the sorts of things that require measurement. These may be as a result of requests from others (such as your manager or professional body) or to support developments for your service users (such as purchasing new equipment or providing new treatments). It may also be that you simply need evidence to support your CPD. Whatever the reason, the following sections will explore some of the aspects that can be measured and how.

What aspects of CPD can you measure?

There are many things you can measure in relation to CPD, depending on your particular role. These aspects are most effectively articulated by answering certain questions. The relevant questions will depend on the nature of the CPD you have undertaken and the context of your work. A few examples are given below.

Questions relating to the impact of your CPD on yourself:

- Has the CPD activity increased my knowledge and skills and influenced my practice?
- In what way has CPD influenced my practice?
- Has my level of confidence changed?

- What, if anything, would I do differently next time?
- Have I met the objectives I set for my CPD? If so, how?
- Can I place a tick against the first four HCPC standards?
- Have I visited every appropriate station for TRAMm?

Questions relating to the impact of your CPD on your service users:
- Has my learning from my CPD activity/ies had an impact (positive or negative) on my service users?
- What specific impact has my CPD had on my service users?
- Are my service user outcomes significantly different since I undertook my CPD activity?
- How has my CPD impacted on the performance or ability of my service users?
- What do my service users think of my intervention?
- Have my peers or colleagues noticed any changes in service user performance?
- What, if anything, would I do differently next time?

Questions relating to the impact of your CPD on your organisation:
- Has my CPD had an impact on service delivery?
- How has my CPD had an impact on service delivery?
- Have I saved my organisation any money?
- Have I generated any income for my organisation?
- Have I influenced organisational strategy through my CPD?
- Has my CPD contributed to policy development?
- What, if anything, would I do differently next time?

Once you have decided on the question you wish to answer, there are various mechanisms that facilitate measurement. The following section gives a brief overview of each.

How do we measure CPD and what can we use as evidence?

In health and social care, the word 'evidence' features regularly and evidence is expected to underpin everything that we do. What do we mean by evidence and how can we distinguish between 'good' and 'bad' evidence?

Researchers generally accept that there is a 'hierarchy of evidence' when evidencing CPD (Burns, Rohrich, et al. 2011). However, while it is useful to consider these issues when evaluating and measuring your CPD, it is important not to get too concerned about the type of evidence; the quality of your evidence is always more important. While a systematic review, based on a meta-analysis of many studies, may be considered the best form of evidence from a research perspective, it may not necessarily be an appropriate way to evaluate an individual's CPD (see also Chapter 9).

For health and care professionals, the HCPC is the regulatory body responsible for setting the standards for CPD (HCPC 2017a) and auditing to ensure that the standards are consistently being met by registrants. You should always have these standards in the forefront of your mind during your CPD process.

If you are one of the 2.5% of registrants selected for audit in any given year (which for each professional group happens biennially), you will be required to renew your registration and submit a profile on a HCPC template. The first section asks you to outline your current role and responsibilities (approximately 500 words) and the second requires you to demonstrate your CPD and how it has met the standards, especially Standards 3 and 4 (no more than 1500 words). This profile should be submitted with evidence, together with a chronological list of all CPD activities and dates undertaken in the last two years (HCPC 2019d). For full details of the HCPC audit process, visit https://www.hcpc-uk.org/.

The HCPC has a range of resources in different formats to help you prepare your documentation if you are selected for audit. Table 10.2 provides HCPC information.

Table 10.2 Useful HCPC information

Information	How to access (website accessed 19.3.2020)
Health and Care Professions Council (HCPC) Continuing Professional Development information	Free downloads available from: https://www.hcpc-uk.org/cpd/ Hard copies available from: Email: publications@hcpc-uk.org
Contact the Health and Care Professions Council (HCPC)	Health and Care Professions Council (HCPC) 184–186 Kennington Park Road, London SE11 4BU https://www.hcpc-uk.org/contact-us/ Tel: +44 (0) 300 500 6184 Email: registration@hcpc-uk.org
Health and Care Professions Council (HCPC) CPD Audit Information	https://www.hcpc-uk.org/cpd/cpd-audits/
HCPC Video presentations on CPD	View on the HCPCuk YouTube channel at: https://www.youtube.com/user/HCPCuk
HCPC sample CPD profiles for each of the registered professions; also check with your individual professional body for more examples and information	Free downloads available at: https://www.hcpc-uk.org/cpd/cpd-audits/completing-a-cpd-profile/how-to-complete-your-cpd-profile/cpd-sample-profiles/

The most important thing to consider when deciding upon your evidence is the connection between what you are measuring or need to evidence and what you are using. For example, if you have been on a course and wish to demonstrate application of CPD in practice (HCPC, Standard 3), a certificate will not suffice on its own. However, the certificate will form part of your evidence to show that various CPD activities have been undertaken (HCPC, Standard 1).

When considering how to evidence what you have achieved through CPD, there are many different methods you can use. Table 10.3 provides an overview of the types of evidence you might wish to consider for each of the HCPC standards and the section that follows explains some of the core methods to help you to decide on an approach to measuring or evidencing your CPD.

Table 10.3 Types of evidence

HCPC standard	Type of evidence	Examples of evidence
1 Record of CPD	Chronological dated list	• TRAMm Tracker • Other CPD record form • Professional Development Portfolio
2 Range of activities	Lists/authenticating documents	• Certificates • Testimonials • TRAMm Trail • TRAMm Tracker • Self-designed list • Online record
3 Application in practice	Reflection	• Written reflection • Extracts from supervision report
	Documentation	• Service evaluation reports • Publications • Research reports • Quality Improvement Project reports • Policy document or strategy highlighting contribution • Case studies
	Service user feedback	• Group or intervention evaluations • Research project/service evaluation • Module/course feedback
	Feedback from manager/other	• Extract from appraisal • Extract from supervision record • Performance indicators • Commendations/professional awards • Accreditations, e.g. fellowships

4 Benefits for service user	Measured outcome	• Outcome measures • Standardised assessments (before and after) • Exam results and report
	Research	• Research reports/peer-reviewed articles
	Service user/carer/feedback	• Anecdotal evidence • Intervention evaluations • Research project data reports • Service evaluation reports
	Student evaluation	• National Student Survey • Module/course/programme evaluations
5 Call for audit	Record of activity	• TRAMm Tracker • Printed on-line record
	Variety of activities	• TRAMm Tracker • TRAMm Trails • Written profile • CPD Profile or Portfolio (if requested)
	Application in practice	• TRAMm Trail • Reflective statement • CPD Profile or Portfolio (if requested)
	Benefit for service users	• Reflective Statement, CPD portfolio (if requested)

Research

Undertaking research is one of the best forms of evidence in terms of application of CPD. In Chapter 2 we looked at research as a CPD activity and the benefits of this for your professional development. Research is considered to be one of the most rigorous means of measurement and there are many different types of research study, depending on the question that needs to be answered. Contrary to popular belief, it is not necessary to undertake large randomised controlled trials if you wish to use research to evidence the impact of your CPD. If this were the case, very few of us would ever attempt to use research in this way. However, it is important that you select the correct methodology and ensure that your study is *ethical*, valid (tests what it is supposed to test) and reliable (the data collection 'tool' you use can produce the same results every time it is used). A small pilot project, which assures validity and reliability and acknowledges limitations, is much more valuable as evidence than a poorly conducted large study.

Firstly, you need to decide if you plan to undertake a research study or whether what you intend is not true research but instead an audit or service evaluation (Health Research Authority 2019). In short, a research study will usually involve the inclusion of something new or a manipulation of variables; an audit will benchmark something against predetermined standards; and a service evaluation is an evaluation of current practice as it stands. Audits and evaluations can still provide valuable evidence of CPD and procedures are often much simpler to follow than if full scientific approval is required. For more comprehensive details, see audits and service evaluations (below) or access the HRA website (https://www.hra.nhs.uk), which has a useful decision-making tool to help you clarify the nature of your study: http://www.hra-decisiontools.org.uk/research/.

If you have never done research before, or have only undertaken a small study as part of your university degree, don't let that put you off but ask for help from someone who understands the process and the pitfalls. In large organisations such as the NHS there are people whose role is to help you with research projects. On the other hand, if you are in a smaller unit or a non-traditional setting, you will need to think about others who may be able to provide research mentorship – for example, staff at your local university or a person who already has a research-based qualification such as a doctorate. You may find that this new partnership is mutually beneficial if the act of being a mentor can contribute towards the other person's CPD.

Collaborative projects are helpful, as a critical eye can often help you avoid some of the biases that may arise, particularly if you are researching something that you have designed or changed yourself. Many get drawn into the trap of trying to 'prove' that what they have done has had a positive impact and this can impede the trustworthiness of the study. Others forget to consider the presence of any confounding variables (such as other treatments, the environment or medication) that may be responsible for the success of the study, rather than the specific intervention that is being researched. Remember, even if a study discovers that what you have introduced has had no impact or a negative impact, it still gives evidence of the application of your CPD in practice and a development in knowledge and/or skills. Admittedly, this may initially be disappointing but may still benefit service users if you stop doing an unhelpful intervention or change how it is done. This is just as important as showing that something works.

Using research to evidence your CPD

As a health and care professional, it is expected that, even if you are not undertaking formal research, you should show how you have used research evidence to support your practice. Investigating and applying research evidence can be considered part of your CPD, but you must record how you have used it in order to demonstrate learning. See Example 10.1 (below).

Example 10.1 Using research as CPD

Imagine that you have attended a one-day course on mindfulness and you decide that this might be a useful intervention for some of your clients who are presenting with depression. You reread the guidance that the trainers have given, regarding the implementation of mindfulness, and then undertake a search to explore whether any systematic reviews or other trustworthy research studies have highlighted specific factors that are essential to its success. (For example, is it best done in a group or on a one-one basis? And how often should people practise it?) You critique the studies to assure yourself that they are valid and reliable. You then map your findings onto an intervention evidence chart (see Table 8.1) to justify your practice and create an evidence file for mindfulness in your department.

Audit

Audit is a crude, yet often useful, measurement of CPD for both the individual and the organisation. At one time, the term 'audit' was invariably associated with money. In healthcare, various audits are now undertaken, such as clinical audit and documentary audit. Audits involve the systematic checking of standards against previously designed benchmarks in order to drive up quality in an organisation or individual.

In an organisation, audits offer an efficient way of providing valuable data regarding improvements in service delivery and associated tasks. For instance, in relation to patient reports, standards are defined and a benchmark percentage stipulated (for example, at least 93% of reports must meet the given standards at 100% accuracy). Following this, all reports are checked against the standards during a specified period. The outcome measure (usually delivered as a percentage of those that fully meet the standard) is then announced and compared with the benchmark percentage. Recommendations may then be made for improvement, and the benchmark percentage may be changed (usually in an upward direction) for the next audit.

In terms of your own CPD, the TRAMm Tracker could be used as your own mini audit. The boxes represent the standards, and the benchmark is set for the percentage of boxes ticked for each CPD activity; or 100% of boxes should be ticked across CPD activities during a specified period of time.

From a manager's or organisation's perspective, audit can also be applied to CPD. In Chapter 9, we discussed a range of suggestions for monitoring CPD, including the various activities undertaken or the number of hours taken by each staff member for CPD. Each of these could be subject to audit separately or they could be combined as a 'CPD audit'. Monitoring these aspects of CPD may include keeping a record through supervision, while an audit will provide an actual measure.

This will be invaluable if you are required to provide reports for the organisation or professional bodies. As a manager, you may find the headings of the TRAMm Tracker useful to structure your audit tool. Alternatively, you may utilise TRAMmCPD to frame CPD within your department, and the audit could be based around staff completion of the Tracker and Trails, with percentage targets for completion of each of the boxes on the chart and numbers of Trails.

Service evaluation

A service evaluation is similar to research, in that you are investigating the impact of something, but the difference here is that you are not changing any of the variables or normal assessment or treatment approaches for the people who access your service or stakeholders. For example, you run a six-week community memory group for patients who have early stage dementia. You always undertake a baseline assessment at the start of the group and redo this at the end of the six weeks. Your evaluation will involve comparing scores before and after and providing a report on the impact of this specific group. The findings will not be generalisable to any other similar group run elsewhere, either within your organisation or across other organisations. We should be carrying this out as part of normal practice but evaluation formalises the process.

The important thing is that you are not doing anything different from what you would normally do for current or new interventions. You use the same criteria for inclusion, you run the same types of sessions, and the assessments you undertake before and after are the same. Occasionally you may decide to measure an intervention (where you are not currently doing so) or introduce a new intervention, but this is what you are required to do as part of professional practice so it is still service evaluation.

Standardised assessments and outcome measures

Outcomes measures are essential in order to measure the impact of an intervention or programme on a service user, stakeholder or service. They are an important part of service delivery for all sectors or professionals who are keen to justify their role. It is important to use standardised assessments or outcome measures exactly as they are designed to be used; this will help to reduce some of the potential flaws in terms of validity. If you design your own assessment tool without piloting, there is a danger that you may get results that do not accurately depict the real outcome. For example, when your service user is discharged, how do you know that this is due to your professional intervention rather than that of the team or another profession?

Grant (1999) highlighted the fact that outcome measures are also important for measuring the impact of professional development, although the process can be complex. Finding measures that evidence the impact of CPD on attitudes and practice requires a different approach from those needed to evidence impact on service users. Measurements of effect on service users are usually based on evaluation tools and professional judgements.

Appraisals/individual performance reviews/professional development reviews

Appraisals are a requirement of most large health and care organisations for all staff and are usually undertaken by a person's line manager once every six to twelve months. In some organisations, appraisals are linked to performance-related pay, but for health and care workers the aim of appraisals is generally to ensure that all staff are developing appropriately according to their level of responsibility and working in line with the strategic direction of the organisation. Having an appraisal system in place also demonstrates the organisation's commitment to professional development.

If carried out correctly, the appraisal process will involve opportunities for review partway through the appraisal period (see Chapter 9). In addition, appraisal should not be used as an opportunity for initial discussions regarding any concerns about performance; these should be highlighted as and when they arise, rather than waiting for a scheduled appraisal. Progress with professional development in relation to concerns previously highlighted may, however, form part of the discussion.

The appraisal process usually focuses on four main areas:

1. Clarifying the main current and aspirational roles of the appraisee
2. Reviewing the objectives set in the previous appraisal, alongside the evidence supporting the appraisee's achievement
3. Identifying any performance limiting or supporting factors in relation to the workplace
4. Setting new objectives for the forthcoming period, together with personal training and development needs.

In order to ensure that the appraisal process works for you and supports or evidences your professional development, it is important to give careful thought to preparing for your appraisal meeting. With this aim in mind, it is useful to take stock of your current roles and responsibilities, reflect upon how they link with your own preferred or aspirational profile, consider your achievements since the last appraisal and summarise your evidence for this. It is also important to carefully consider your future objectives and training or development needs. When you put these together you must ensure that:

- The objectives are written using a SMART format to enable you to have non-contested discussions as to whether or not they have been achieved (see Chapter 4)
- The objectives give due consideration to the strategic direction of your department and wider organisation
- At least one or two objectives are related to the application of CPD and having a direct or indirect impact on service users or stakeholders
- At least one objective should include how you plan to disseminate the impact of your CPD with those who have invested in your learning
- The objectives reflect (in part or in full) your aspirations for professional development. Even if you do not intend to do everything in the forthcoming period, it is useful to begin to 'hint' about your aspirations. For example, you may not wish to start a Masters degree this year but you may identify and record an objective in your appraisal/PDR to investigate possible areas for research.

Measuring informal learning

Informal learning occurs when you least expect it. It may be something that is explained or debated in the staffroom, a discussion over lunch with a colleague, an observation made in the community or an incident or issue via a television programme. This learning is no less valuable even though it can be difficult to measure or assess (Mathers, Mitchell & Hunn 2012). If you wish to evidence this, the most effective option is to undertake a written reflection that identifies the source of the learning, what it has helped you to understand and how this learning has influenced or will influence your practice and/or benefit your service users or stakeholders.

Preceptorship

In Chapter 9 we introduced the concept of preceptorship and how it can be used to monitor progress. Preceptorship can also be a mechanism for measurement, as successful progress through individual professional development plans linked to the Knowledge and Skills Framework (KSF) leads to incremental advance. Successful achievement of preceptorship offers measurable evidence that you have reached the standard required for working in that organisation.

Records are kept throughout preceptorship to provide evidence that the process has occurred and that CPD has taken place. These records can then be used to provide the evidence required to sign-off on final completion. A similar process in other organisations, called 'probation', usually occurs for a defined period of time (around 12–36 months); during this time the individual has regular meetings with a line manager who is responsible for overseeing the individual's professional development. Successful completion of probation can lead to a full contract of employment and/or a higher pay band.

Peer review and measurement

As we saw in Chapter 9, peer review can take many forms and can either make up part of the monitoring process or provide a way of measuring CPD. Although some aspects of peer review provide a measurement of organisational progress, they can also be used as evidence of your own performance. Examples of this are given below.

One type of summative peer review is self-regulation by qualified members of a profession from the same field. An example of this might be accreditation in healthcare education, normally every five years, where any degree programme leading to a professional award is subject to review by colleagues to ensure its fitness for the award it is conferring. During this process, formative feedback may be offered but there is also an outcome, in terms of whether the programme is approved. This may involve commendations, conditions (which must be addressed) and/or recommendations (which must be given consideration). At the end of the process, a final decision is taken as to whether the professional body is happy to accredit the programme for a further specified period of time.

Another type of summative peer review assesses suitability for publication (e.g. in a journal or book) or presentation (e.g. at a conference). In this instance, the outcome or measurement is the decision as to whether or not the work is accepted. Taking part in peer review can be considered a CPD activity, whether you are the reviewee or reviewer, and the outcome of the review can provide valuable evidence regarding your professional development.

For example, you have led a programme review and preparation of documentation for accreditation, and the organisation receives feedback that the new programme presented demonstrates innovation and full team engagement in the planning. You could then use this as evidence of your developing leadership ability, and it may also be used as evidence of achievement of one of your outcomes set at appraisal. Likewise, if a paper you have written is accepted for publication, you could use this as evidence of your ability to undertake research or measurement in terms of disseminating your CPD.

Measurements required by organisations

In 2006, the World Health Organisation described six dimensions defining quality, where improvement should continually be sought. One of these was the need for care to be efficient (maximising resources and avoiding waste). At a macro level, organisations are not only interested in the success of your CPD benefiting the service as a whole but also the cost-effectiveness of such intervention. There is limited evidence to support the cost-effectiveness of CPD. However, the alternative to CPD, the implementation of unsupported interventions, could be considered a wasteful use of resources in itself.

Quality-adjusted life years (QALYs) are defined and described by the National Institute for Health and Care Excellence (NICE 2019) as:

> A measure of the state of health of a person or group in which the benefits, in terms of length of life, are adjusted to reflect the quality of life. One QALY is equal to 1 year of life in perfect health. QALYs are calculated by estimating the years of life remaining for a patient following a particular treatment or intervention and weighting each year with a quality of life score (on a zero to 1 scale). It is often measured in terms of the person's ability to perform the activities of daily life, freedom from pain and mental disturbance.

QALYs may therefore offer a useful unit of measurement if you are attempting to demonstrate the cost-effectiveness of a specific intervention designed during CPD, but experience is required with their use, so it is recommended that advice is sought before you consider utilising them.

In most cases it is probably more appropriate to measure how much money your CPD has cost. You can then balance this information against, for example, discharge times versus cost of hospital beds per day, money saved on staff time if procedures have been streamlined, or income generated versus the cost of undertaking CPD. Your manager, finance or research department should be able to help you consider ways in which these comparisons can be most effectively calculated.

For those of us providing health and/or social care, it is impossible to avoid risk altogether and people may occasionally undergo treatments or interventions where there is the potential for harm. However, people have a right to expect care from skilled and knowledgeable staff who can help them decide what is best in their case. Safety should be a core focus for any organisation. Any CPD where application of learning may help to increase the safety of people accessing the service is therefore considered important. This impact must be measurable in some way, though it is not always easy to link it to CPD.

Safety can be measured both quantitatively and qualitatively. Using quantitative methodologies often involves setting targets and measuring compliance – for example, incident reporting, or cases of infection, following an audit approach. The National Advisory Group on the Safety of Patients in England (NAGSPE 2013) highlights the limitations of this approach in certain instances (such as reporting incidents) where non-reporting or inaccurate reporting leads to inaccurate data. Instead, Brown and Lilford (2008) advocate the use of a mixed methods approach in order to both define problems and measure impact.

Measurement may take the form of research or evaluations, and these quality improvement projects are often useful to address issues affecting the safety of people who access services. Subsequent reports can provide excellent evidence of CPD in relation to HCPC Standards 3 and 4.

Using informal or anecdotal evidence

Formal types of evidence are easier to produce, but it is often informal anecdotal evidence from service users that provides us with the most immediate feedback. However, it is difficult to know how to use anecdotal evidence, particularly if you are selected for the HCPC audit. So how do we use and record anecdotal material as evidence?

Some types of anecdotal evidence may be abstract aspects, such as time or confidence. Your reflections may reveal that you feel more confident undertaking a skill or activity, or you realise that you have become much quicker at completing what was once a more time-consuming task. Conversely, as you become more confident in using a new skill, the task may take longer as you are able to become less procedural, more relaxed and able to converse. Feedback from others can help increase confidence in your learning.

Before you start using anecdotal evidence, remember that you are bound by your professional body and the HCPC to respect confidentiality when reporting anything. If you are ever unsure about the necessity of this, err on the side of caution and do not use names or any other significant identifying features.

There are several ways to do this, as listed in Table 10.4 below.

The contents of the table could also be captured in your reflections and documented as anonymised quotes to support what you are saying.

Table 10.4: Referencing anecdotal evidence

Type of evidence	How to capture NB: All need to be anonymised versions for submission (HCPC 2017d).
Conversation with service users/carers/students' feedback	Document this in case notes, or have it recorded in supervision or appraisal records
Confidence or time taken to perform a task/skill	Reflect on how your confidence has increased and the time taken to perform the task/skill has decreased
Emails	Anonymise first, then print off the email/s
References or testimonials	Request permission from the provider and submit permission with the document
Feedback via social media	Take screenshots, use on-line information collation and/or digital curation tools (see Chapters 6, 7 and 8), anonymised as appropriate
Text feedback	Screenshot (and either digitally anonymise or remove identification) and photocopy
Cards/Letters of thanks	Anonymise first, then photocopy/print

Using TRAMmCPD to measure CPD

Some examples of how the TRAMm Tracker and Trail can be used to measure or evidence CPD have been identified above and details of their completion are given in Chapter 7.

The TRAMm Tracker has been designed to be used as an 'at-a-glance' record of engagement in CPD, which can be submitted as your CPD record during the HCPC audit process. It is easy to identify CPD undertaken, and where there is potential for further development. The TRAMm Tracker enables you to record formal and informal activities carried out and identify any gaps in terms of maintaining or reaching HCPC standards or missing visits to TRAMm stations.

Although the TRAMm Trail does not provide any specific measurement, it offers a more detailed summary of the more significant activities and station visits. They can be completed fairly quickly, as a reminder of the evidence you have, or the evidence you still need to collect.

From the feedback we have had from the pilot evaluation, people have found it most effective to use their TRAMm Tracker and TRAMm Trail as 'works in progress', updating them as they go along. They have used them in their supervision sessions and annual appraisals to highlight what has been achieved and identify their learning needs. TRAMmCPD can help you identify your learning needs by highlighting the gaps and encouraging you to consider how they can be addressed. The decision as to which TRAMm station each element of CPD fits into is entirely subjective, although suggestions are included as to what might be appropriate in each chapter.

This also applies to meeting the HCPC CPD standards (see Example 10.2). When deciding on the appropriate TRAMm station for a particular element of your CPD, it is important to consider the following questions:

1. How does this TRAMm station or HCPC standard relate to the specific aspect of learning and CPD?
2. Can you justify why it fits into the TRAMm station/s or under the HCPC standard/s?
3. What evidence can you produce to support this?

Example 10.2 Does supervision meet all the HCPC standards?

Question from practitioner: In the TRAMmCPD information available on your website, it states that supervision only covers HCPC Standards 1 and 2. However, I would argue that supervision covers all four standards. Here are my reasons.

Practitioner justification – HCPC Standard 1:
Yes, completing my TRAMm Tracker demonstrates that I am maintaining a continuing, chronological, up-to-date and accurate record of my CPD activities.
TRAMmCPD mentor response: Yes, I agree.

Practitioner justification – HCPC Standard 2:
Yes, my TRAMm Tracker demonstrates I am carrying out a mixture of learning activities.
TRAMmCPD mentor response: Yes, I agree.

Practitioner justification – HCPC Standard 3:
Yes, by participating in supervision, I am ensuring that my CPD has contributed to the quality of my practice.
TRAMmCPD mentor response: Not necessarily. Where is your evidence to show that your supervision session has considered the application of your CPD specifically, rather than normal work practice? If you can justify how, then you can tick this box.
(See Chapters 5 and 7 for discussion regarding when normal work becomes CPD.)

Practitioner justification – HCPC Standard 4:
Yes, regular supervision obviously benefits my service users through discussion of their needs and my interventions.
TRAMmCPD mentor response: Not necessarily. Talking about it and doing it are two different things. Firstly, are your discussions reflective, critical and suggesting action points? Or are you just having a chat about your normal work practice? Where is your evidence to show that you have learnt something from the supervision that is contributing to your CPD, that you have applied it in practice and there has been an impact on your service user/s? (See Chapters 6 to 10.)

Bear in mind that not all your learning experiences will address all the TRAMm stations. This should not be a matter for concern – as long as you are visiting all stations deemed appropriate over time, can justify why others are not appropriate, and can ensure that you visit all stations across the range of CPD you undertake.

Case study: Sally collates evidence for her portfolio

Sally is an occupational therapist. Over the last two years, she has progressed from being complacent about CPD to becoming fully engaged in the process, using TRAMmCPD as her guide. She has now developed a sound CPD portfolio, which is easy to access, and she has evidence in case she is called for HCPC audit or is required to complete any applications for future posts in her field. She has completed rotation posts in the areas of orthopaedics, mental health and neurorehabilitation, and she is about to finish her fourth rotation in rheumatology. She is hoping that a Band 6 position in the field of neurorehabilitation will soon become available. In the meantime, she is continuing with activities to develop her skills and profile across all four Pillars of Practice within the occupational therapist's career development framework (RCOT 2017).

Sally meets the occupational therapy manager for her first proper appraisal since she started this post and completed her preceptorship 12 months ago. They review the objectives she set 12 months ago and Sally begins to realise how much has changed in her approach to CPD, her professionalism and her knowledge and skills since her final preceptorship review.

Using her TRAMm Tracker and TRAMm Trails to frame her discussion, she highlights the CPD she has measurements for, and presents her evidence to her line manager as follows:

She has learnt about and jointly presented TRAMmCPD to the multidisciplinary team. **Evidence:** In relation to application and benefit to users of TRAMmCPD, Sally produces her TRAMm Trail and talks through the CPD activities she has undertaken that have had a positive impact on her practice. She also shows the manager some feedback she has had following the presentation she did for her peers. She notes that four of them are now using TRAMmCPD and have set up a TRAMmCPD support group, with Sally as the main facilitator.

She has a certificate for the two-day training course she undertook on CBT and has been applying the principles. She is aware that if she wishes to use this as a focused intervention, she will need to undertake the full training and is currently considering this. **Evidence:** Anecdotal, comprising positive verbal feedback received from her neurorehabilitation mentor, which has been explicitly documented in Sally's supervision record, which she shows to her line manager. She also has a reflection based upon her work with a student and the learning resource she developed as a result, which students and new starters have commended as invaluable.

Sally has now undergone a day's training in the driving assessment centre, following which she has designed, written and implemented a 'return to driving after stroke pathway'. **Evidence:** A clear, concise, written pathway for returning to driving following neurological deficit; a case study that illustrates a patient's experience when following the pathway. She has presented this work at her employer's annual best practice conference and has received a quality improvement award for excellent innovative practice. Sally has already submitted an abstract to present at the professional annual conference.

Her manager highlights the enormous progress Sally has made this year, which has included achievements over and above the objectives set the previous year. They discuss and agree new objectives for the coming year, and Sally's manager says she will happily support any applications Sally makes for Band 6 positions in the future.

Tasks

1. Consider the measurement tools you currently know about or use in your work, and think about how they could be used to measure aspects of your own CPD.

2. Make a note for your next appraisal or performance review to ensure that your objectives are SMART and contain at least one objective that relates to the application of your planned CPD.

3. Consider a specific question you wish to answer and identify an appropriate methodology by which to measure it. Decide if this is research, audit or service evaluation.

4. Consider ways in which you could use your CPD to make cost savings for your organisation, or how you might use it to generate some income. Think about how you might show the cost-effectiveness of your CPD in either situation.

5. Complete the measurement section for at least one TRAMm Trail and consider the measurements you may already have for the specific activity and your plans to measure in the future.

6. Update your TRAMm Tracker.

7. Consider how you will share the impact of one piece of your CPD with your organisation.

8. Read Chapter 11 to understand the key messages from each chapter in this book.

How do you measure your CPD? TRAMm Station m: measure

Figure 10.1 Sally's updated TRAMm Tracker

Date	Activity description	Certificate	Reflection	TRAMm Trail	HCPC Standards					TRAMm				Index	Notes
					1	2	3	4	5	T	R	A	M	m	
DD/MM/YY	Service development – Design new return to driving pathway	C	R	T	1	2	3	4		T	R	A	M	m	4/5	See TRAMm Trail: Service development; attendance certificate and quality improvement award stored in CPD file
DD/MM/YY	Career Development Planning – Current skills mapped to Career Development Framework		R	T	1	2				T	R	A	M	m		See TRAMm Trail: Career Development Planning and SWOT Analysis
DD/MM/YY	Self-directed learning – Rotation into neurorehabilitation		R	T	1	2	3	4		T	R	A	M	m		See TRAMm Trail: Rotation into Neurological Rehabilitation; stored on CPD memory stick
DD/MM/YY	Preceptorship		R		1	2	3	4		T	R	A	M	m		All documentation stored in Preceptorship file
DD/MM/YY	Introduced to TRAMmCPD by a colleague in a staff meeting			T	1	2	3	4		T	R	A	M	m	3	Learning about TRAMmCPD, organised and presented information to team colleagues. Details in TRAMmCPD TRAMm Trail

A Strategic Guide to Continuing Professional Development for Health and Care Professionals:
THE TRAMm Model

TRAMm Trail

Please note: The TRAMm Trail has been designed for you to plan and record in a little more depth your most significant pieces of CPD. It is not anticipated that you will complete this for every piece of your CPD; only those you feel may be useful for evidence if called by the HCPC for audit. Please ensure that you maintain confidentiality.

Figure 10.2 Sally's TRAMm Trail: Service development

TRAMm Trail: Service Development – Return to Driving Pathway Following Stroke Date: DD/MM/Y

TELL (T)	RECORD (R)	APPLY (A)
• Informal discussions with manager of the ABI Team for advice when consultants have requested inappropriate assessment of patients (DD/MM/YY – ongoing) • Provided verbal feedback to the Team Leader, In-Patient Therapy Lead and Therapy Services Manager about existence of the Rookwood Driving Battery and potential benefit to our service (DD/MM/YY – ongoing) • Informally discussed plans for returning to driving pathway with Stroke Association (DD/MM/YY) • Verbal feedback to patients re: concerns about the impact of cognitive deficits on their ability to return to driving (DD/MM/YYs) • Post questions on social media to see what others have set up or are already doing (DD/MM/YY) • Meet with Senior Occupational Therapist to start pathway and feedback progress to Therapies Manager	• CPD certificate of attendance from training event (DD/MM/YY) (Index 3 in CPD file) • Reflection using Fish and Twinn (1997); Strands of Reflection completed from fitness to drive training stored on USB stick (DD/MM/YY) • Rookwood record forms completed and filed in patient notes (DD/MM/YY) • Feedback to GPs and consultants with results and concerns in patients' discharge letters (DD/MM/YY) • Case notes documented in patients' notes (DD/MM/YY) • TRAMm Trail initiated (DD/MM/YY) and updated (ongoing), to be used in annual appraisal • Collated record of social media interactions (DD/MM/YY) • Supervision records (DD/MM/YY) • Clear concise written pathway for returning to driving following neurological deficit • TRAMm Tracker (DD/MM/YY)	• Integrated all training, evidence and knowledge to design a return to driving pathway (DD/MM/YY) • Undertaken return to driving assessments (DD/MM/YY)

MONITOR (M)	mEASURE (m)	HCPC Standards met: 1, 2, 3, 4
• Informal supervision with Team Manager to support progress and monitor pathway progression (DD/MM/YY) • Formal supervision with Senior OT (DD/MM/YY); discussed increasing the use of Rookwood Battery within the service (DD/MM/YY) • Self-monitoring using Fish and Twinn (1997); Strands of Reflection (DD/MM/YY) • Pathway trialled and outcomes discussed with Team Manager before final pathway agreed (DD/MM/YY)	• Improved service to patients, with clear concise written pathway for returning to driving following neurological deficit (DD/MM/YY) • Case study completed to illustrate patient journey/experience when following driving pathway (DD/MM/YY) • Return to driving pathway service development successfully implemented, demonstrating increasing leadership skills (DD/MM/YY) • Quality improvement award received from excellent practice; Certificate stored in CPD Portfolio Index 4 (DD/MM/YY)	**PLAN of ACTION** • *Feedback to Stroke Unit therapists, Stroke consultants and Stroke Association* • *Present at national annual professional conference (abstract submitted DD/MM/YY)* • *Update Reflection* • *Update TRAMm Tracker and Trail*

164

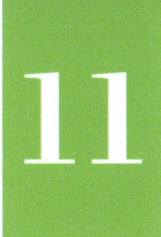

Conclusion

Continuing professional development is a personal journey. This handbook has been written and updated for health and care professionals to illustrate the use of the **TRAMm Model** and its tools, the **TRAMm Tracker and TRAMm Trail (TRAMmCPD)**, while also providing a comprehensive guide to encourage your strategic engagement in **CPD** (Hearle & Lawson 2019). The key messages from each chapter are summarised below.

Chapter 1: What is continuing professional development (CPD) and why do we do it?

In this chapter we explored the nature of CPD, and why we must engage in it as health and social care professionals.

Key messages

- As a health and social care professional, CPD is mandatory and is regulated by the HCPC.
- CPD is your responsibility as a professional but can be facilitated by a number of people as well as your organisation.
- In order to demonstrate your engagement in CPD, you must show its application in practice and its impact on yourself and others according to the HCPC Standards for CPD (HCPC 2017a).
- There are a number of organisations you can contact (both national and international) for information and advice about CPD in other countries.

Chapter 2: What counts as CPD activity?

Any activity from which you learn and develop can be used to further your professional development.

Key messages

- Engaging in any form of activity can be effective if it is suited to your particular strengths and learning needs.
- Individuals often engage in activities that contribute towards their professional development without realising that they are potentially undertaking CPD.

- When planning your CPD, ensure the activities you select benefit you, your organisation and your service users and are recorded in your TRAMm Tracker and TRAMm Trail.
- CPD activities do not have to cost money; there are many that are freely available.

Chapter 3: Taking responsibility for CPD: Changing mindsets

Here we explored the nature of CPD engagement and your individual responsibilities in relation to fully engaging in the learning and development process.

Key messages

- There are five defining attributes of CPD engagement.
- CPD engagement can occur despite a lack of physical resources or time.
- A proactive approach to CPD is invaluable.
- There are a range of frameworks to enable you to map your learning and development.

Chapter 4: Recognising and developing your preferred learning style

Understanding your strengths and preferred learning styles, and addressing your CPD in a way that reflects them, may help you to engage with it more effectively.

Key messages

- CPD is a personal journey and there is no such thing as 'one size fits all'.
- There are various tests and activities available that can help you identify your preferred learning style and ways to maximise learning opportunities.
- For CPD to be most effective, identifying your strengths and preferred learning needs, and articulating these objectively, can help ensure that they are measurable.

Chapter 5: Introduction to the TRAMm model

This chapter introduced mechanisms for strategic CPD using TRAMmCPD.

Key messages

- Doing CPD is not the same as engaging in CPD.
- CPD is important for job satisfaction and quality of practice and its impact on service users.
- TRAMmCPD consists of a model to guide your approach, and tools (TRAMm Tracker and Trail) to record and track your progress.
- TRAMmCPD can help you plan and execute appropriate professional development to meet your needs, along with those of your service users and the organisation in which you work.

Conclusion

Chapter 6: How do you plan and disseminate your CPD? TRAMm Station T: TELL

Communication is a vital part of CPD, which helps you to plan and disseminate your learning so that it can be effective and benefit others.

Key messages

- Planning is essential. It can be formal or informal and goals may be strategic or designed for the short term.
- Plans should not be concrete but, instead, fluid and adaptable to change.
- Creating your own learning communities can help your engagement in CPD and maintain your professional identity.
- Disseminating your learning is your professional responsibility.
- There are many ways to disseminate information, depending on your preference and the information you wish to impart.

Chapter 7: How do you record your CPD plans and activities? TRAMm Station R: RECORD

This chapter explored why it is important to document your CPD and different mechanisms you can use to record your CPD.

Key messages

- Various recording mechanisms are available to suit your individual preference, including written, visual, verbal and virtual media.
- The TRAMm Tracker provides a continuous record of CPD undertaken.
- The TRAMm Trail provides greater depth of information regarding specific areas of learning, which can be used for planning and recording your CPD.
- The TRAMm Trail can provide an immediate prompt for your reflections.
- Both the TRAMm Tracker and TRAMm Trail may be used as part of your submission for HCPC audit.

Chapter 8: How can you apply your learning? TRAMm Station A: Apply

Applying your learning in practice is an essential prerequisite of being a health and care professional and explicit within the HCPC standards for CPD (HCPC 2017a).

Key messages

- It is important to use your new knowledge and skills in practice to benefit yourself, your service users, your team, organisation and others.
- You need to consider the appropriateness of, and evidence for, what you have learnt before using it in practice.
- TRAMmCPD can help you keep track of how you have applied your learning and who has benefitted.

Chapter 9: How do you keep track of your CPD? TRAMm Station M: MONITOR

It is essential to monitor your progress in order to ensure that your professional development is a continuous journey.

Key messages

- Self-monitoring is vital. It involves taking stock of what you have achieved and considering your short- and long-term aspirations.
- Ways of monitoring CPD include supervision, mentorship, preceptorship, peer review, annual appraisal and reflection.
- It is important to document the monitoring progress and outcomes.
- The TRAMm Tracker and Trail can be used to monitor your progress and facilitate progress discussions.

Chapter 10: How do you measure your CPD? TRAMm Station m: mEASURE

The outcomes and impact of your CPD can be measured in a variety of ways and this provides evidence to indicate your progress and future direction.

Key messages

- TRAMmCPD encourages an output measurement approach, focused on the way you apply and use your learning.
- Planning and setting specific goals provide you with a baseline from which to measure the success of your CPD.
- The TRAMm Tracker and TRAMm Trail measure your performance in relation to HCPC standards and TRAMm stations.
- TRAMmCPD can help you structure your evidence if you are selected for HCPC audit.
- CPD is a continuous journey and it is important to share the impact of your learning with others (Chapter 6 – TELL).

Conclusion

All these key messages have been incorporated within each chapter through our continuous case study, where we have used TRAMmCPD to illustrate Sally's progressive engagement in the concept of CPD.

Continuing the CPD journey

You should now have a clear understanding of how to engage in your learning and development, the HCPC requirements for CPD and how to use TRAMmCPD to help you develop a strategy to advance your personal and professional journey over the next 12 months – and the next 5–10 years.

Our own journey continues, as we further develop TRAMmCPD, and we welcome your queries and feedback. Research is ongoing, and further updates will be made to TRAMmCPD as our studies progress.

Good luck on your CPD journey and remember that the latest information and TRAMmCPD tools are free to download from www.TRAMmCPD.com

References

Academy of Medical Royal Colleges (AMRC) (2010). *The Effectiveness of Continuing Professional Development (Final Report).* London: General Medical Council.

Allied Health Professions Project (AHPP) (2003). *Allied health professions project: Demonstrating competence through CPD.* https://webarchive.nationalarchives.gov.uk/+/http://www.dh.gov.uk/en/Consultations/Closedconsultations/DH_4071458 (Accessed 22 March 2020).

Alsop, A. (2013). *Continuing Professional Development in Health and Social Care. Strategies for Lifelong Learning.* 2nd edn. Chichester: Wiley-Blackwell. ISBN: 978-1-118-53956-9

Bargagliotti, A.L. (2012). Work engagement in nursing: a concept analysis. *Journal of Advanced Nursing.* **68**(6), 1414–28. doi.org/10.1111/j.1365-2648.2011.05859.x.

Barry, M., Kuijer-Siebelink, W., Nieuwenhuis, L. & Scherpbier-de Haan, N. (2017). Communities of practice: A means to support Occupational Therapists' Continuing Professional Development. A literature review. *Australian Occupational Therapy Journal.* **64**(2), 185–93. doi: 10.1111/1440-1630.12334 10.1111/1440-1630.12334.

Berndt, A., Murray, C., Kennedy, K., Stanley, M. & Gilbert-Hunt, S. (2017). Effectiveness of distance learning strategies for Continuing Professional Development (CPD) for rural allied health practitioners: A systematic review. *BMC Medical Education.* **17**(117), 1–13. doi.org/10.1186/s12909-017-0949-5.

Billett, S. (2001). Learning through work: Workplace affordances and individual engagement. *Journal of Workplace Learning.* **13**(5), 209–14. doi:10.1108/EUM0000000005548.

Bodell, S. & Hook, A. (2011). Using Facebook for professional networking: a modern-day essential. *British Journal of Occupational Therapy.* **74**(12) 588–90. doi:10.4276/030802211X13232584581533.

Bodell, S., Hook, A., Penman, M. & Wade, W. (2009) Creating a learning community in today's world: How blogging can facilitate Continuing Professional Development and international learning. *British Journal of Occupational Therapy.* **72**(6), 279–81.

Borko, H., Mayfield, V., Marion, S., Flexer, R. & Cumbo, K. (1997). Teachers' developing ideas and practices about mathematics performance assessment: Successes, stumbling blocks, and implications for professional development. *Teaching and Teacher Education.* **13**, 259–78. doi.org/10.1016/S0742-051X(96)00024-8.

Boud, D. (1988). *Developing Student Autonomy in Learning.* London: Routledge, Kegan Paul.

Boud, D. & Middleton, H. (2003). Learning from others at work: Communities of practice and informal learning. *Journal of Workplace Learning.* **15**(5), 194–202. doi:10.1108/13665620310483895.

Boyer, S.L., Edmondson, D.R., Artis, A.B. & Fleming, D. (2013). Self-directed learning: A tool for lifelong learning. *Journal of Marketing Education.* **36**(1), 20–32. doi:10.1177/0273475313494010.

Brangan, J., Quinn, S. & Spirtos, M. (2015). Impact of evidence-based practice course on Occupational Therapists' confidence levels and goals. *Occupational Therapy in Health Care.* **29**(1), 27–38. doi:10.3109/07380577.2014.968943.

Brown, C. & Lilford, R. (2008). Evaluating service delivery interventions to enhance patient safety. *British Medical Journal.* **337**: a2764. doi.org/10.1136/bmj.a2764.

Broughton, W. & Harris, G. (eds) on behalf of the Interprofessional CPD and Lifelong Learning UK Working Group (2019). *Principles for Continuing Professional Development and Lifelong Learning in Health and Social Care.* Bridgwater: College of Paramedics.

Burbank, M. & Kauchak, D. (2003). An alternative model for professional development: investigations into effective collaboration. *Teacher and Teaching Education.* **19**(5), 499–514. doi.org/10.1016/S0742-051X(03)00048-9.

Burns, B.P., Rohrich, R.J., & Chung, K.C. (2011). The levels of evidence and their role in evidence-based medicine. *Plastic and Reconstructive Surgery.* **128**(1), 305–10. doi: 10.1097/PRS.0b013e318219c171.

Canadian Institutes of Health Research (CIHR) (2005). *Developing a CIHR framework to measure the impact of health research* (CIHR synthesis report). https://www.researchgate.net/publication/253670933_A_framework_to_measure_the_impact_of_investments_in_health_research (Accessed 22 March 2020).

Care Quality Commission (CQC) (2013). *Supporting information and guidance: Supporting effective clinical supervision.* London: Care Quality Commission.

Chartered Society of Physiotherapy (CSP) (2017). *Clinical supervision: a brief overview.* https://www.csp.org.uk/publications/clinical-supervision-brief-overview (Accessed 22 March 2020).

College of Occupational Therapists (COT) (2010). *Management briefing, supervision.* London: COT.

College of Occupational Therapists (COT) (2015). *Supervision for Occupational Therapists and their Managers.* London: COT.

Constable, G. (2013). 'Reflection as a catalyst in the development of personal and professional effectiveness' in D. Blogg & M. Challis (eds) *Evidencing CPD: A Guide to Building Your Social Work Portfolio.* Northwich: Critical Publishing. 53–69.

Critical Appraisal Skills Programme (CASP) (2019). *CASP Checklists: Making Sense of Evidence.* https://casp-uk.net/casp-tools-checklists/ (Accessed 24/11/19).

Cusick, A. & McCluskey, A. (2000). Becoming an evidence-based practitioner through professional development. *Australian Occupational Therapy Journal.* **47**, 159–70. doi:10.1046/j.1440-1630.2000.00241.x.

Dall'Alba, G. (2009). Learning professional ways of being: Ambiguities of becoming. *Educational Philosophy and Theory.* **41**(1), 34–45 doi:10.1111/j.1469-5812.2008.00475.x.

Dall'Alba, G. & Barnacle, R. (2005). Embodied knowing in online environments. *Educational Philosophy and Theory.* **37**, 719–44. doi:10.1111/j.1469-5812.2005.00153.x.

Dall'Alba, G. & Sandberg, J. (2006). Unveiling professional development: A critical review of stage models. *Review of Educational Research.* **76**(3), 383–412. doi:10.3102/00346543076003383.

Davies, C.H.F. III., Regina Deli-Amen, R., Rios-Aguilar, C. & Gonzalez Canche, M.S. (2012). Social media in higher education: A literature review and research directions. Arizona: University of Arizona and Claremont Graduate University.

Davis, D., Evans, M., Jadad, A., Perrier, L., Rath, D., Ryan, D., Sibbald, G., Straus, S., Rappolt, S., Wowk, M. & Zwarenstein, M. (2003). The case for knowledge translation: shortening the journey from evidence to effect. *British Medical Journal.* **327**, 33–35. doi.org/10.1136/bmj.327.7405.33.

Delors, J. (1996). *Learning: The Treasure Within.* Paris. UNESCO. http://www.unesco.org/education/pdf/DELORS_E.PDF (Accessed 22 March 2020).

Department of Health (DH) (1998). *The New NHS: Modern, Dependable.* London: The Stationery Office.

Department of Health (DH) (2001). *Our Healthier Nation: A Contract for Health.* London: The Stationery Office.

Department of Health (DH) (2002). *Learning from Bristol: The Department of Health's Response to the Report of the Public Inquiry into Children's Heart Surgery at the Bristol Royal Infirmary 1984–1995.* https://www.gov.uk/government/uploads/system/uploads/attachment_data/file/273320/5363.pdf (Accessed 22 March 2020).

Department of Health (DH) (2004). *Agenda for Change Final Agreement.* http://webarchive.nationalarchives.gov.uk/20130107105354/http://www.dh.gov.uk/en/Publicationsandstatistics/Publications/PublicationsPolicyAndGuidance/DH_4095943 (Accessed 22 March 2020).

Department of Health (DH) (2010). *Preceptorship Framework for Newly Registered Midwives, Nurses and AHPs.* https://www.networks.nhs.uk/nhs-networks/ahp-networks/documents/dh_114116.pdf (Accessed 22 March 2020).

Desimone, L.M. (2009). Improving impact studies of teachers' professional development: Toward better conceptualizations and measures. *Educational Researcher.* **38**(3), 181–99.

Dixon-Woods, M. (2010). Why is patient safety so hard? A selective review of ethnographic studies. *Journal of Health Services and Research Policy.* **15**(1), 11–16.

Edmondson, D.R., Boyer, S.L. & Artis, A.B. (2012). Self-directed learning: A meta-analytic review of adult learning constructs. *International Journal of Education Research.* **7**(1), 40–48.

Edmonson, A. & Moingeon, B. (1998). From organizational learning to the learning organization. *Management Learning.* **29**(1), 5–20. doi:10.1177/1350507698291001.

Fish, D., & Twinn, S. (1997). *Quality Supervision in the Health Care Professions. Principled Approaches to Practice.* Oxford: Butterworth-Heinemann.

Fleming, N.D. & Mills, C. (1992). Not another inventory, rather a catalyst for reflection. *To Improve the Academy.* **11**, 137–55.

Foucault, M., Vachon, B., Thomas, A., Rochette, A. & Giguere, C.E. (2017). Utilisation of an electronic portfolio to engage rehabilitation professionals in continuing professional development: results of a provincial survey. *Disability and Rehabilitation.* **40**(13), 1591–1600. doi:10.1080/09638288.2017.1300335.

Frank, J.R., Snell, L.S., Cate, O.T., Holmboe, E.S., Carraccio, C., Swing, S.R., Harris, P., Glasgow, N.J., Campbell, C., Dath, D., Harden, R.M., Lobst, W., Long, D.M., Mungroo, R., Richardson, D.L., Sherbino, J., Silver, I., Taber, S., Talbot, M. & Harris, K.A. (2010). Competency-based medical education: theory to practice. *Medical Teacher.* **32**(8), 638–45. doi: 10.3109/0142159X.2010.501190.

Friedman, A. (2012). *Continuing Professional Development: Lifelong Learning of Millions.* Abingdon: Routledge.

Garvin, D.A., Edmondson, A.C. & Gino, F. (2008) Is yours a learning organization? *Harvard Business Review.* 1–17. https://hbr.org/2008/03/is-yours-a-learning-organization (Accessed 22 March 2020).

Gibbs, G. (1988). *Learning by Doing: a Guide to Teaching and Learning Methods.* Oxford Further Education Unit.

Gibbs, V. (2011). An investigation into the challenges facing the future provision of Continuing Professional Development for Allied Health Professionals in a changing healthcare environment. *Radiography.* **17**, 152–57. doi:10.1016/j.radi.2011.01.005.

Gopee, N. (2015). *Mentoring and Supervision in Healthcare.* 3rd edn. London: Sage Publications Ltd.

Gould, D., Drey, N. & Berridge, E.J. (2007). Nurses' experiences of continuing professional development. *International Journal of Nursing Studies.* **27**(6), 602–609. doi: 10.1016/j.nedt.2006.08.021.

Grant, J. (1999). Measurement of learning outcomes in continuing professional development. *The Journal of Continuing Education in the Health Professions.* **19**, 214–21.

Great Britain (2018). *Data Protection Act.* London: The Stationery Office.

Gunn, H. & Goding, L. (2009). Continuing Professional Development of physiotherapists based in community primary care trusts: a qualitative study investigating perceptions, experiences and outcomes. *Physiotherapy.* **95**, 209–214. doi: 10.1016/j.physio.2007.09.003.

Halle, M., Mylopoulos, M., Rochette, A., Vachon, B., Menon, A., McCluskey, A., Amari, F. & Thomas, A. (2018). Attributes of evidence-based Occupational Therapists in stroke rehabilitation. *Canadian Journal of Occupational Therapy.* **85**(5), 351–64. doi.org/10.1177/0008417418802600.

Haywood, H., Pain, H., Ryan, S. & Adams, J. (2012). Engagement with Continuing Professional Development: Development of a service model. *Journal of Allied Health.* **41**(2), 83–89.

Haywood, H., Pain, H., Ryan, S. & Adams, J. (2013). Continuing Professional Development: Issues raised by nurses and allied health professionals working in musculoskeletal settings. *Musculoskeletal care.* **11**, 136–44. doi.org/10.1002/msc.1033.

Health and Care Professions Council (HCPC) (2015). *Preventing Small Problems from Becoming Big Problems in Health and Social Care.* London: HCPC.

Health and Care Professions Council (HCPC) (2016). *Standards of Conduct, Performance and Ethics.* London: HCPC.

Health and Care Professions Council (HCPC) (2017a). *Continuing Professional Development and Your Registration.* London: HCPC.

Health and Care Professions Council (HCPC) (2017b). *Guidance on Social Media.* London: HCPC.

Health and Care Professions Council (HCPC) (2017c). *Confidentiality – Guidance for Registrants.* London: HCPC.

Health and Care Professions Council (HCPC) (2019a) *Professions and Protected Titles* https://www.hcpc-uk.org/about-us/who-we-regulate/the-professions/ (Accessed 22 March 2020).

Health and Care Professions Council (HCPC) (2019b). *Continuing Professional Development Audit Report 2015–2017.* London: HCPC.

Health and Care Professions Council (HCPC) (2019c). *Benefits of Becoming a Reflective Practitioner. A Joint Statement of Support from Chief Executives of Statutory Regulators of Health and Care Professionals.* London: HCPC.

Health and Care Professions Council (HCPC) (2019d). *How to Complete your Continuing Professional Development Profile.* https://www.hcpc-uk.org/cpd/cpd-audits/completing-a-cpd-profile/how-to-complete-your-cpd-profile/ (Accessed 22 March 2020).

Health Education England (HEE) (2019). *Preceptorships.* https://www.hee.nhs.uk/our-work/preceptorships (Accessed 22 March 2020).

Health and Safety Executive (HSE) (2019). *Work-related stress, anxiety or depression statistics in Great Britain, 2019.* https://www.hse.gov.uk/statistics/causdis/stress.pdf (Accessed 22 March 2020).

Health Foundation (2010). *Evidence Scan: Complex Adaptive Systems.* London: The Health Foundation.

Health Research Authority (HRA) (2019). *What approvals do I need?* https://www.hra.nhs.uk/approvals-amendments/what-approvals-do-i-need/ (Accessed 22 March 2020).

Hearle, D., Lawson, S. & Morris, R. (2016). *A Strategic Guide to Continuing Professional Development for Health and Care Professionals: The TRAMm Model.* Keswick: M&K Publishing.

Hearle, D. & Lawson, S. (2019). Continuing Professional Development (CPD) engagement – a concept analysis. *Journal of Continuing Education in the Health Professions.* **39**(4), 251–59. doi:10.1097/CEH.0000000000000245.

Honey, P. & Mumford, A. (1992). *The Manual of Learning Styles.* Maidenhead: Peter Honey.

Holdsworth, L., Douglas, D., Hunter, E. & McDonald, C. (2013). Social media: Raising the profile of AHPs. *British Journal of Healthcare Management.* **19**(2), 85–92.

Hughes, K. (2018). The use of Twitter for Continuing Professional Development within Occupational Therapy. *Journal of Further and Higher Education.* **44**(1), 113–25. doi: 10.1080/0309877X.2018.1515900.

Illing, P.J., Crampton, P., Rothwell, C., Corbett, S., Tiffin, P. & Trepel, D. (2017). *What Is the Evidence for Assuring the Continuing Fitness to Practise of Health and Care Professions Council Registrants, Based on Its Continuing Professional Development and Audit System?* Newcastle: Newcastle University.

Intensive Care Society (2018). *Allied Health Professions Critical Care Professional Development Framework.* https://www.ics.ac.uk/ICS/Resources___AHP_Framework.aspx (Accessed 22 March 2020).

Jamieson, L., Harris, L. & Hall, A. (2012). Providing support for newly qualified practitioners in Scotland. *Nursing Standard.* **27**(2), 33–36. doi: 10.7748/ns2012.09.27.2.33.c9296.

Johns, C. (1994). Nuances of reflection. *Journal of Clinical Nursing.* **3**, 71–75. doi.org/10.1111/j.1365-2702.1994.tb00364.x.

Johnson Coffelt, K. & Gabriel, L. (2017). Continuing competence trends of Occupational Therapy practitioners. *The Open Journal of Occupational Therapy.* **5**(1), 1–17. doi:10.15453/2168-6408.1268.

Kavanagh, D.J., Spence, S.H., Strong, J., Wilson, J., Sturk, H. & Crow, N. (2003). Supervision practices in allied mental health: Relationships of supervision characteristics to perceived impact and job satisfaction. *Mental Health Services Research.* **5**, 187–95. doi:10.1023/A:1026223517172.

Knowles, M.S. (1975). *Self-Directed Learning. A Guide for Learners and Teachers.* Englewood Cliffs: Prentice Hall/Cambridge.

Kolb, D.A. (1984). *Experiential Learning: Experience as the Source of Learning and Development.* New Jersey: Prentice-Hall.

Krätzig, G.P., & Arbuthnott, K.D. (2006). Perceptual learning style and learning proficiency: A test of the hypothesis. *Journal of Educational Psychology.* **98**(1), 238–46. doi.org/10.1037/0022-0663.98.1.238.

Lawson, S. (2018). *Occupational Therapists Understanding of and Engagement in Continuing Professional Development.* Belfast: Royal College of Occupational Therapists Annual Conference and Exhibition.

Lawson, S. & Hearle, D. (2019a). A lifelong journey. *OTNews.* **27**(1), 30–31.

Lawson, S. & Hearle, D. (2019b). *The Application of Learning for CPD.* Birmingham: Royal College of Occupational Therapists Annual Conference and Exhibition.

Lawson, S. & Tempest, S. (2019). *Learning Communities for CPD.* Royal College of Occupational Therapists Annual Conference and Exhibition. Birmingham.

Learning and Skills Research Centre (2004). *Learning styles and pedagogy in post-16 learning – a systematic and critical review.* https://www.voced.edu.au/content/ngv%3A13692 (Accessed 22 March 2020).

Legare, F., Borduas, F., MacLeod, A., Sketeris, I., Campbell, B. & Jacques, A. (2011). Partnerships for knowledge translation and exchange in the context of continuing professional development. *Journal of Continuing Education in the Health Professions.* **33**(3), 181–87. doi: 10.1002/chp.20125.

Lloyd, B., Pfeiffer, D., Dominish, J., Reading, G., Schmidt, D., & McCluskey, A. (2014). The New South Wales allied workplace learning study: barriers and enablers to learning in the workplace. *BMC Health Services Research.* **14**(134), 1–17.

Lowe, M., Rappolt, S., Jaglal, S. & Macdonald, G. (2007). The role of reflection in implementing learning from continuing education into practice. *Journal of Continuing Education in the Health Professions.* **27**(3), 143–48. doi.org/10.1002/chp.1340240108.

Maclean, F., Jones, D., Carin-Levy, G. & Hunter, H. (2013). Understanding twitter. *British Journal of Occupational Therapy.* **76**(6), 295–98. doi:10.4276/030802213X13706169933021.

Marsick, V. & Watkins, K. (2015). *Informal and Incidental Learning in the Workplace.* London: Routledge.

Maslach, C., Schaufeli, W. B. & Leiter, M. (2001). Job burnout. *Annual Review of Psychology.* **52**, 397–422.

Mathers, N., Mitchell, C. & Hunn, A. (2012). *A Study to Assess the Impact of Continuing Professional Development (CPD) on Doctors' Performance and Patient/Service Outcomes for the GMC.* Sheffield: The University of Sheffield in collaboration with Capita Health.

McClelland, D.C. (1985). How motives, skills and values determine what people do. *American Psychologist.* **40**, 812–25.

Mol, A. (2002). *The Body Multiple: Ontology in Medical Practice.* Durham, NC: Duke University Press.

Moon, J.A. (2004). *A Handbook of Reflective and Experiential Learning: Theory and Practice.* London: Routledge Falmer.

Moorley, C. & Chinn, T. (2015). Using social media for continuous professional development. *Journal of Advanced Nursing.* **71**(4), 713–17.

Murray, K. & Ward, K. (2017). Attitudes to social media use as a platform for Continuing Professional Development (CPD) within Occupational Therapy. *Journal of Further and Higher Education.* 1–16. doi:10.1080/0309877X.2017.1378313.

Myers, C., Schaefer, N. & Coudron, A. (2017). Continuing competence assessment and maintenance in Occupational Therapy: Scoping review with stakeholder consultation. *Australian Journal of Occupational Therapy.* **64**, 486–500. doi:10.1111/1440-1630.12398.

National Advisory Group on the Safety of Patients in England (NAGSPE) (2013). *A promise to learn – a commitment to act: Improving the Safety of Patients in England.* London: Williams Lea. https://www.gov.uk/government/uploads/system/uploads/attachment_data/file/226703/Berwick_Report.pdf (Accessed 22 March 2020).

National Institute of Care and Excellence (NICE) (2019). *Glossary*. https://www.nice.org.uk/glossary?letter=q (Accessed 22 March 2020).

NHS (2019). *The NHS Long Term Plan*. https://www.longtermplan.nhs.uk/publication/nhs-long-term-plan/ (Accessed 22 March 2020).

NHS Education for Scotland (2012). *Pillars of Practice*. http://www.careerframework.nes.scot.nhs.uk/using-the-framework/pillars-of-practice.aspx (Accessed 22 March 2020).

NHS Employers (2016). *A Social Media Toolkit for the NHS*. https://www.nhsemployers.org/-/media/Employers/Publications/Social-media/Social-Media-Toolkit.pdf (Accessed 22 March 2020).

NHS Staff Council (2009). *Improving Working Lives in the NHS – A Framework Developed by the NHS Staff Council*. London: NHS Employers.

Newton, P.M. & Miah, M. (2017). Evidence-based higher education – is the learning styles 'myth' important? *Frontiers in Psychology*. **8**, 444. doi: 10.3389/fpsyg.2017.00444.

Nursing and Midwifery Council (NMC) (2019). *Revalidation: How to Revalidate with the NMC*. London: NMC.

Oakes, J. & Rogers, J. (2007). Radical change through radical means: Learning power. *Journal of Educational Change*. **8**, 193–206. doi:10.1007/s10833-007-9031-0.

O'Keeffe, C. (2016). Book Reviews: A Strategic Guide to Continuing Professional Development for Health and Care Professionals: The TRAMm Model. *Nursing Management*. **23**(2), 16.

Olinky, E. (2009). *Clinical Supervision in Occupational Therapy, Burnout and Related Phenomena*. https://library.iated.org/view/OLINKY2011CLI (Accessed 22 March 2020).

O'Neill, E. (2004). *Professional Supervision: Myths, Culture and Structure*. Co. Tipperary: RMA Publications.

O'Sullivan, J. (2003). Unlocking the workforce potential: is support for effective continuing professional development the key? *Research in Post-Compulsory Education*. **8**(1), 107–22. doi:10.1080/13596740300200143.

O'Sullivan, J. (2006). 'Continuing Professional Development' in R. Jones & F. Jenkins (eds) *Developing the Allied Health Professional*. Oxford: Radcliffe Publishing. 1–16.

Øvretveit, J. (2009). *Does Improving Quality Save Money? A review of the evidence of which improvements to quality reduce costs to health service providers*. London. Health Foundation.

Øvretveit, J. (2011). Understanding the conditions for improvement: research to discover which context influences affect improvement success. *BMJ, Quality and Safety*. **20**(1), i18–i23.

Oxford Paperback Dictionary and Thesaurus (2007). 2nd edn. Oxford: Oxford University Press.

Parsloe, E. & Leedham, M. (2009). *Coaching and Mentoring: Practical Conversations to Improve Learning*. 2nd edn. London: Kogan Page.

Penman, M. (2014). *Do we have what it takes? An investigation into New Zealand occupational therapists' readiness to be self-directed learners*. https://oatd.org/oatd/record?record=handle%5C%3A10523%5C%2F4596 (Accessed 22 March 2020).

Playfoot, J. & Hall, R. (2018). *The Future of Learning in the Workplace. The Transformative Power of Collaborative Social Learning* [Online]. Future Learn. https://www.futurelearn.com/workplace-learning/whitepaper (Accessed 22 March 2020).

Poulsen, A., Meredith, P., Khan, A., Henderson, J., Castrisos, V. & Khan, S. (2014). Burnout and work engagement in Occupational Therapists. *British Journal of Occupational Therapy*. **77**(3), 156–64. doi: 10.4276/030802214X13941036266621.

Rickles, D., Hawe, P. & Shell, A. (2007). A simple guide to chaos and complexity. *Journal of Epidemiology and Community Health*. 61, 933–37. doi:10.1007/978-3-030-28018-5_2.

Rodgers, C. (2002). Seeing student learning: Teacher change and the role of reflection. *Harvard Educational Review*. **72**(2), 230–53.

Rolfe, G., Freshwater, D. & Jasper, M. (2001). *Critical reflection in nursing and the helping professions: a user's guide*. Basingstoke: Palgrave Macmillan.

Royal College of Nursing (RCN) (2007). *Joint Statement on Continuing Professional Development for Health and Social Care Practitioners*. London: RCN.

Royal College of Occupational Therapists (RCOT). (2017) *Career Development Framework: Guiding Principles for Occupational Therapy*. London: Royal College of Occupational Therapists.

Rushton, H., Gorry, G., Stanley, K., Sorlie, C. & Murray, K. (2016). Social media: Creating communities of research and practice. *British Journal of Occupational Therapy*. **79**(4), 195–96. doi:10.1177/0308022616631551.

Ryan, J. (2003). Continuous Professional Development along the continuum of lifelong learning. *Nurse Education Today*. **23**, 498–508. doi:10.1016/S0260-6917(03)00074-1.

Scally, G. & Donaldson, L.J. (1998). Clinical governance and the drive for quality improvement in the new NHS in England. *British Medical Journal*. **317**(7150), 61–65. doi.org/10.1136/bmj.317.7150.61.

Schaufeli, W.B. & Bakker, A.B. (2004). Job demands, job resources, and their relationship with burnout and engagement: a multisample study. *Journal of Organizational Behavior.* **25**, 293–315. doi:10.1002/job.248.

Schon, D.A. (1983). *The Reflective Practitioner: How Professionals Think in Action.* London: Temple Smith.

Silversides, K. (2015). *Perceptions and Experiences of the HCPC Approach to Continuing Professional Development Standards and Audits: Report for the HCPC.* York: Qa Research.

Simpson, M.R. (2009). Engagement at work: A review of the literature. *International Journal of Nursing Studies.* **46**(7), 1012–24. doi:10.1016/j.ijnurstu.2008.05.003.

Skills for Care (2019). *Developing Social Workers.* https://www.skillsforcare.org.uk/Learning-development/social-work/Developing-social-workers.aspx (Accessed 22 March 2020).

Straus, S.E., Tetroe, J. & Graham, I. (2009). Defining knowledge translation. *Canadian Medical Association Journal.* **181**(3–4), 165–68. doi:10.1503/cmaj.081229.

Strong, J. (2009). 'Clinical supervision skills' in E.A.S. Duncan (ed) *Skills for Practice in Occupational Therapy.* London: Churchill Livingstone. 338–49.

Strong, J., Kavanagh, D., Wilson, J., Spence, S., Worrall, L. & Crow, N. (2003). Supervision practice for allied health professionals within a large mental health service: Exploring the phenomenon. *The Clinical Supervisor.* **22** (1), 191–210. doi: 10.2147/JMDH.S84557.

Taylor, M.C. (2014). Occupational Therapy: Is it evidence-based, evidence-informed or evidence-inspired? *British Journal of Occupational Therapy.* **77**(8), 130. doi:10.1177/030802261407770S804.

Treseder, R. (2012). 'The future of the profession' in T. Polglase & R. Treseder (eds) *The Occupational Therapy Handbook: Practice Education.* Keswick: M&K Update Ltd. 131–48.

Turner, M. (2014). *Evidence-Based Practice in Health.* https://canberra.libguides.com/evidence (Accessed 22 March 2020).

Vachon, B., Foucault, M.L., Giguere, C.E., Rochette, A., Thomas, A. & Morel, M. (2018). Factors influencing acceptability and perceived impacts of a mandatory eportfolio implemented by an Occupational Therapy regulatory organisation. *Journal of Continuing Education in the Health Professions.* **38**(1), 25–31 doi: 10.1097/CEH.0000000000000182.

Van den Broeck, A., Vansteenkiste, M., DeWitte, H. & Lens, W. (2008). Explaining the relationships between job characteristics, burnout and engagement. *Work and Stress.* **22**(3), 277–94.

VARK Questionnaire (2019). http://vark-learn.com/the-vark-questionnaire/ (Accessed 22 March 2020).

Waite, M. & Keenan, J. (2010). *CPD for Non-Medical Prescribers: A Practical Guide.* Chichester: Wiley Blackwell.

Wang, C.L. & Ahmed, P.K. (2003). Organisational learning: a critical review. *The Learning Organization.* **10**(1), 8–17.

Webster-Wright, A. (2009). Reframing Professional Development Through Understanding Authentic Professional Learning. *Review of Educational Research.* **79**(2), 702–739. doi:10.3102/0034654308330970.

Welch, A. & Dawson, P. (2006). Closing the gap: Collaborative learning as a strategy to embed evidence within Occupational Therapy practice. *Journal of Evaluation in Clinical Practice.* **12**(2), 227–38. doi:10.1111/j.1365-2753.2005.00622.x.

Welsh Government (2019). *A Healthier Wales: Our Plan for Health and Social Care.* London: Crown Copyright.

World Health Organisation (WHO) (2006). *Quality of Care: A process for making strategic choices in health systems.* Geneva: WHO.

Youngstrom, M.J. (2009). 'Supervision' in E.B. Crepeau, S.E. Cohn, E.S. Boyt & B.A. Shelle (eds) *Willard & Spackman's Occupational Therapy.* 11th edn. Philadelphia: Wolters Kluwer, Lippincott, Williams & Wilkins. 929–48.

Index

application of learning *119, 120, 121, 122*
application of learning, barriers to *120*
application of learning, demonstration of *124*
appraisals 154, 155
audiovisual aids *84, 85*
audit *149, 152, 153*
blogs, see *weblogs*
clinical governance *2, 3*
clinical supervision *133, 135*
coaching *19*
collaboration *41*
conferences *22, 80, 81–86*
conferences, applying to *83*
conferences, preparing for *84*
confidentiality *93, 158*
continuing professional development (CPD),
    definition of *1*
    courses *23*
CPD activities *11, 12, 13*
CPD, approaches to *61*
CPD, demonstration of *4, 8*
CPD, developing a business case for *46, 47*
CPD engagement *35, 36, 37, 59*
CPD in normal work practice *40, 41*
CPD, international requirements for *6, 7*
CPD, motivating/driving factors *33, 34*
CPD, reasons for undertaking *2, 3*
CPD standards *5*
CPD, undertaking *8*
CPD, what counts as *11–30*
dissemination *71, 79–91*
dissemination, formal *80*
dissemination, informal *79*
education, formal *14, 15*
evidence, informal or anecdotal *158, 159*
evidence, types of *148, 150*
Honey and Mumford learning styles *55*
impact factor *86*
individual performance reviews   154
informal learning, measuring   156
innovative technology presentations   *82*
in-service training   *89*
intervention evidence chart   *124*

journal clubs *17, 18*
journals, peer-reviewed *86*
keynote lecture *81*
knowledge translation *123*
Kolb Learning Style Inventory *54*
learning and development frameworks *38*
learning community *72*
learning contracts *95, 97*
learning culture *43, 44, 45*
learning organisations *45, 60*
learning styles *51–57*
lifelong learning *2, 122*
measurements required by organisations *157*
measuring CPD *145–164*
measuring CPD, methods *148*
measuring CPD, reasons for *146*
mentorship *19, 136*
mind maps *95*
monitoring CPD *129–144*
monitoring CPD, value of for individual *130*
monitoring CPD, value of for organisation *131*
Need for Achievement (nAch) Test *51*
non-verbal skills *85*
online interactions, recording evidence of *99*
organisational learning theory *44, 45*
outcome measurement *146, 154*
peer review *138, 156*
planning *71, 72–79*
planning, formal *75*
planning, individual factors in *75*
planning, informal *74*
planning, organisational factors in *76*
portfolios, CPD *96, 97, 98, 99*
posters *81, 82*
preceptorship *19, 137, 156*
presentations *81*
professional bodies *4*
professional development reviews *154*
professional development, stages of *35*
professional responsibility *3, 32*
professional/external activities *18, 19*
project work *14, 15*
publication, writing for *86, 87*

quality-adjusted life years (QALYs) *157*
recording CPD *93–118*
reflection *28, 29, 94, 137*
reflective logs *94*
regulatory bodies *3*
research *13, 15, 151, 152*
resources *77*
roadshows *88*
round table discussions *83*

self-directed approach *55*
self-directed learning *27, 28, 32*
self-monitoring *137*
seminars *83*
service evaluation *152, 154*
service user, definition of *147*
SMART objectives *56, 73*
social media *25, 26, 27, 87, 88, 100*
standardised assessments *154*
Station A: Apply *65, 66, 119–128*
Station m: measure *65, 66, 145–164*
Station M: Monitor *65, 66, 129–144*
Station R: Record *65, 93–118*
Station T: Tell *65, 71–91*
stress *3*
supervision *19, 46, 133*
support, informal *24, 41*
support, professional *19, 20, 41, 42*
SWOT analysis *141*

talking to others *71*
training *20, 21*
TRAMm Model stations *64, 65*
TRAMm Model, introduction to *59–70*
TRAMm Tracker *63, 66, 68, 101, 102, 103, 111, 112, 138*
TRAMm Trail *63, 66, 67, 101, 102, 105, 106, 113, 114, 138*
TRAMmCPD, reasons to use *67*
TRAMmCPD, using to measure CPD *159*

VARK test *53*
verbal skills *85*

weblogs *100*
work-based learning *16, 17*
workshops *23, 82*